How to Be a Goth

Notes on Undead Style

Tish Weinstock

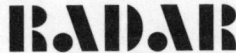

First published in Great Britain in 2024 by Radar, an imprint of
Octopus Publishing Group Ltd
Carmelite House
50 Victoria Embankment
London EC4Y 0DZ
www.octopusbooks.co.uk

An Hachette UK Company
www.hachette.co.uk

The authorised representative in the EEA is Hachette Ireland, 8 Castlecourt
Centre, Castleknock Road, Castleknock, Dublin 15, D15 YF6A, Ireland

ISBN 978-1-80419-236-8

A CIP catalogue record for this book is available from the British Library.

Typeset in 10.75/16pt Farnham Text by Jouve (UK), Milton Keynes

Printed and bound in Great Britain.

13 5 7 9 10 8 6 4 2

This FSC® label means that materials used for
the product have been responsibly sourced.

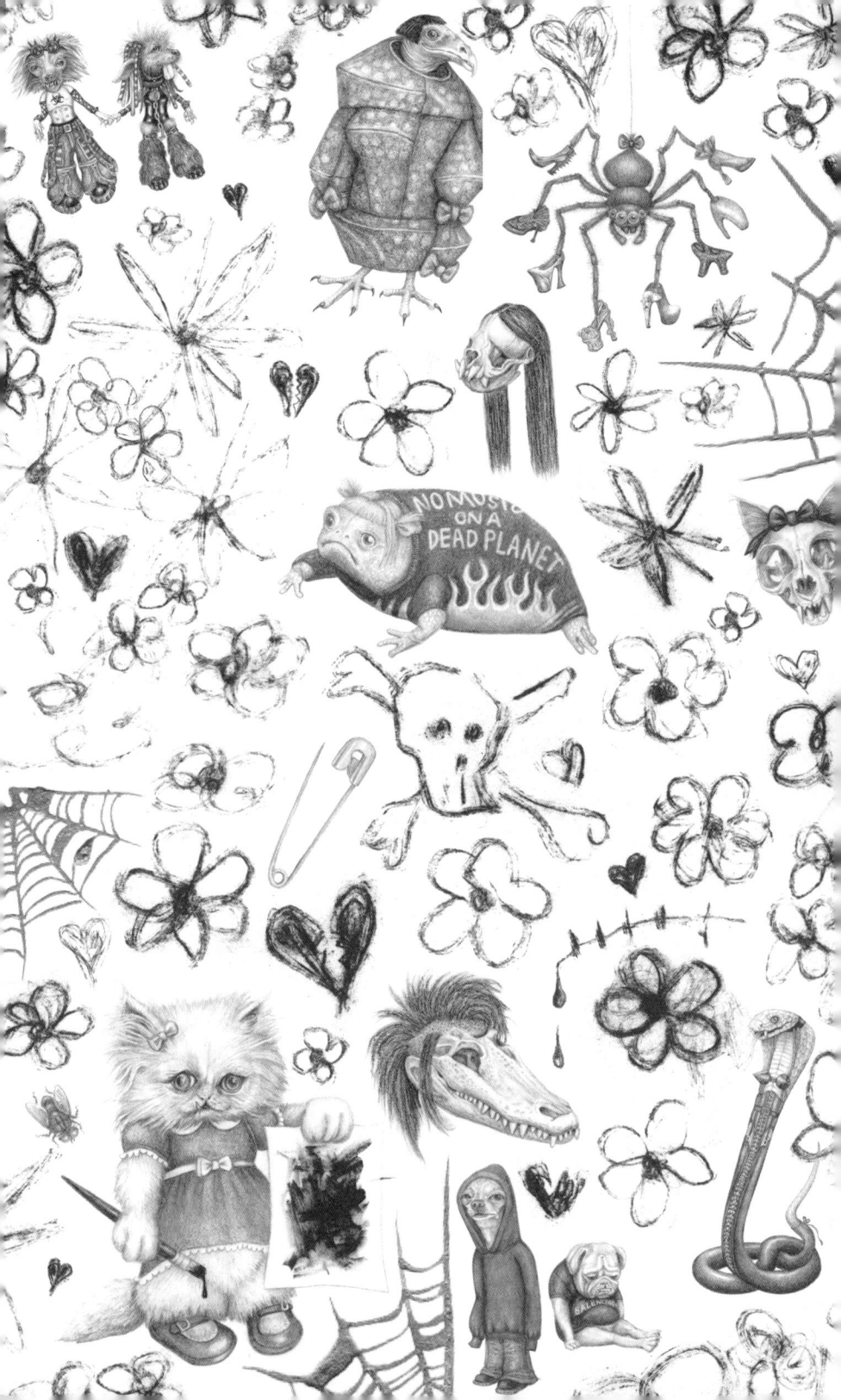

How to Be a Goth

This book is for the misfits, mischief-makers
and miscreants.

Contents

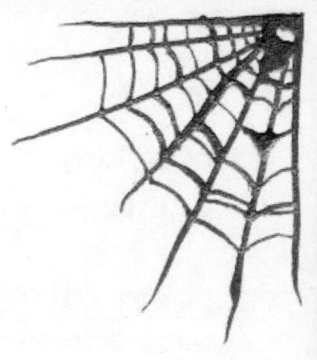

CONTENTS

Preface

Amanda Harlech: notes on black

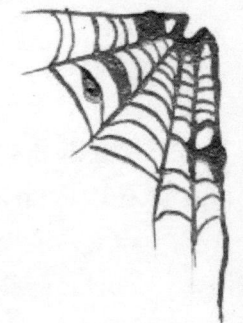

Black defines. Cormorant arrowing low above the winter-light river. Black seeks no approval but withdraws from the commerce of colour like a widow among a plough of pews retreating into shadow. It does not distract, but focuses the eye like belladonna dropped in an iris. Black is rarely as black as [Anish] Kapoor's blackest black, Vantablack, but an eigengrau of achromatic shades of blackness. It is like a silence that still rings with a reverberation of sound long after your ear has stopped hearing the song.

Absence	Ash
Shadow	Jet
Charcoal	Pitch
Ink	Melanin
Payne's Grey	Clinker
Obsidian	

This is the shadowland of my wardrobe – fragile slips of black tulle; stark, scalpel-defined couture tailoring; a ballgown of washed duchess satin that hovers like a memory from a curtain pole. I have always loved the dark edges of things, the melancholy, liminal entre chien et loup, where what might be shivers just out of sight. Wearing black is the key to privacy like the night, allowing me thoughtspace without the distraction of daylight's detailed compulsion. I like to walk in the gloaming. I believe in ghosts, in the portal at the axis of a line of yews where the laurel moves imperceptibly and something shifts, silent as a fox. The quietness of black lets me see feelingly, unobtrusively, without tripping over myself. I admit to being haunted by memories, the ghosts of experiences that drift through us like smoke or the salt of fear.

My great aunt Anne was a miniaturist among a gregarious family of artists. She wore black velvet in mourning for the suffering of so many women. She smoked opium, inhabiting the shadows of her studio like a wraith illumined by candlelight, painting her miniatures with a hair of a hare. She was, according to my mother, mostly silent but as courageous a suffragette as her sisters. Complex as a Chinese perfume bottle painted from the inside, she leads me back into myself when I come home from the bright lights of the photographic studio or the forensic scrutiny of fittings. Wearing black is like feeling my way in the dark, but really feeling, with all my sense tuned up.

Black is white and white is black. They both shine and define. Black – or historically, BHLEG or BHEL – meaning to burn, gleam, flash, bleach; blank, blond, blaze. Black devours the whole visual spectrum, reflecting nothing back, but consuming every visible wavelength until it brims with colour – every colour imaginable. By wearing black you become a distillation, the paint strokes of Sesshu Toyo's *Splashed Ink Landscape* (1495), an austere abstinence from desirous, passionate colour in the drive for a truth – the truth, say, in the grace and economy in the leap of a cat (a black cat), or Gabrielle Chanel's Ford dress. Renaissance black. Black in all its shades is far from negative, it is as positive as white. They exist because of each other, like day and night. I love black for its infinite colour, its powerful ascetic choice and for the way it allows me to be myself.

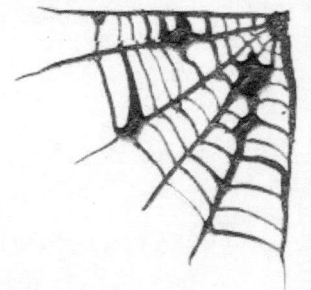

Introduction

The season of the witch

What does it mean to be a goth today? There is, of course, no definitive answer, and it would be reductive to try and provide one. The true aim of this book is to excavate the roots of, and show my aeonian appreciation for, this most hallowed of all subcultures. It will also shed light on those shadowy individuals throughout the ages who have been touched in some way by the codes of goth, holding them up as examples for future goths to draw inspiration from.

The pain of simply existing is something we can all relate to, which is why the state of being goth traverses time and space. An outward expression of otherness, there are myriad ways to be a goth; it's a (life-long) journey of self-discovery.

But why do I sit, now, quill in hand? Growing up, I felt somewhat ashamed of my gothic sensibilities, and it's only as I reached adulthood that I grew the confidence to truly embrace them. And beyond that, as we enter a new apocalyptic era, there's simply no better time to be a goth.

Even before its subcultural inception, the spirit of goth perforated culture at every level: we've seen gothic art, architecture and literature. Since time immemorial, people have filled their stories with sinister characters and spectres of evil as a way to make sense of this harrowing and at times unyielding world. It speaks to some primordial predilection for and preoccupation with darkness, which perhaps accounts for why in the last century, out of all the post-war subcultures – skinheads, punks, mods, rockers, teddy boys – goths form the only tribe that has really endured, albeit cast ever further in the shadows.

Fast-forward to today, however, and goth has done the unthinkable. After years of lingering in the cultural wilderness, thanks to the increasingly dark times in which we now find ourselves, coupled with unprecedented live-streamed access to culture as it happens, goth has finally come crashing into the mainstream.

Those who gravitate towards dark matter tend to possess a somewhat melancholic disposition, a state of being where nothing fits, which can be incredibly isolating. So allow this grimoire to be your companion as you move through the abyss – a manual from which the modern goth may draw encouragement whenever the lure – and pressures – of cultural conformity get too much.

Scythed into the three main stages of a woman's sartorial evolution, *How to Be a Goth* will steer you from cradle to crypt, as you navigate those blistering teenage years, turbulent mid-life crises and final witchy winters. Also thrown into the cauldron is a collection of loose guides that cover everything from what to watch, listen to and read, to how to furnish a home (haunted or otherwise), as well as notes from distinguished vixens across art, fashion, music and film, including model Amelia Gray, actress Anjelica Huston and artist Michèle Lamy, who share what it means to be goth or goth-coded. There's also a letter from demonic duo Fecal Matter about how to scare the mainstream and whimsical illustrations from artist Aurel Schmidt peppered throughout. Elsewhere, there's an inventory of important undead icons through the ages, from Wednesday Addams, Siouxsie Sioux and Theda Bara to Edith Sitwell, Rei Kawakubo and Miss Havisham. Which can only mean one thing: must be the season of the witch.

Chapter I:
Confessions of a goth

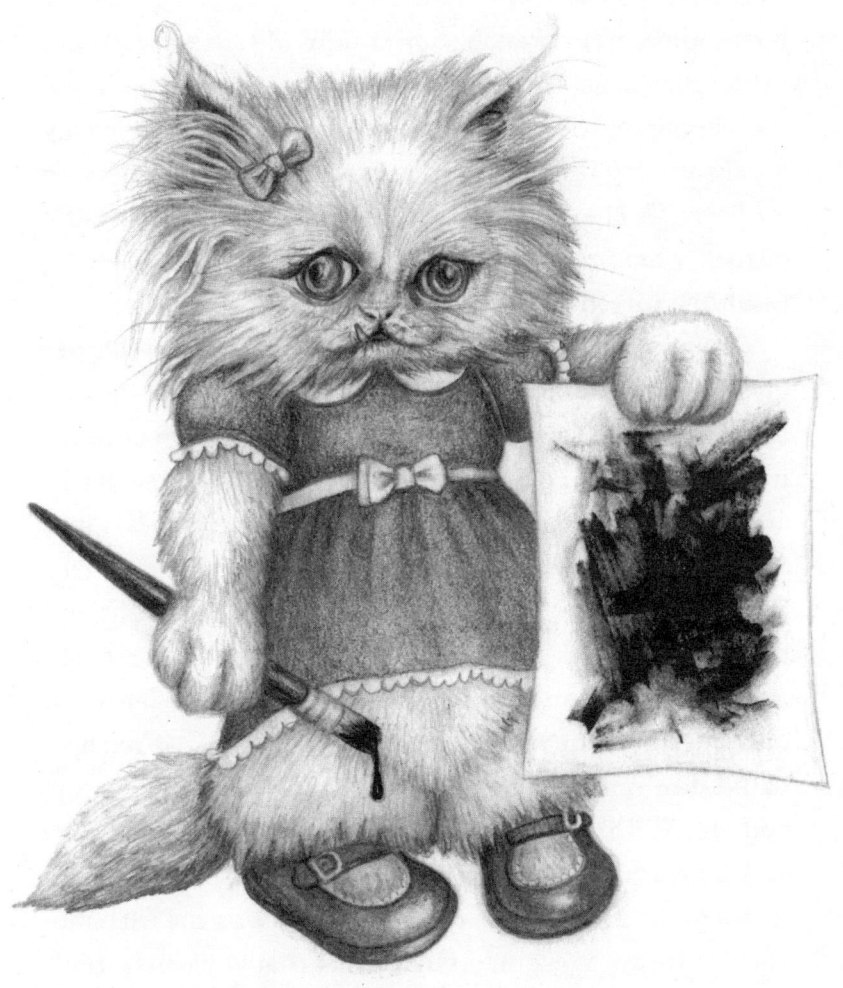

My story starts somewhere in the 90s. I grew up in a listless household in London where precious objects and curious antiques lined the walls of cordoned-off rooms that children weren't allowed to go in. Mausoleum-like, it had been that way since my father died after I turned five. Death hung over our home, infecting every nook and cranny. My sisters were sent to boarding school and my mother took to her tower of grief. A creeping sense of loneliness and discomfort pervaded my youth, as if my skin was permanently crawling. I remember the first time I heard the song *Spaceman* by Babylon Zoo (1996) on the TV music show *Top Of The Pops*, aged six, and something inside me stirred.

Growing up, I wasn't like other kids, those bonnie blonde girls in their pink satin party dresses, preferring instead to wear frocks in red and crushed black velvet. I was never interested in being a princess, either, instead finding an affinity with vampires, ghosts, witches and ghouls. I was about 11 when Morticia Addams entered my orbit via Barry Sonnenfeld's film *The Addams Family* (1991). Brought into being by Anjelica Huston, this deathly apparition made a lasting impression on my young psyche – her jet-black bias-cut silhouette with its eerie tendrils; her blood-red lips, pallid skin and raven hair. She was dark, dangerous, vampy and cool. With my own pale complexion and bitter-chocolate locks, I was drawn to this woman who refused to conform to normative standards of beauty. She was the ultimate gothic pin-up, a testament to the fact that you can be both hot and sad at the same time. Even our nicknames were the same: Tish.

2

By the time my teenage years whipped round, a storm was brewing. And from then on, I became a goth. It wasn't an overnight decision, or even a conscious one, but a progression galvanized by some subconscious attraction to the dark side. At odds with the cultural establishment, I nursed my growing pains with all things macabre. I pored over films like *Edward Scissorhands* (1990), *The Wicker Man* (1973), *The Doom Generation* (1995), *Ghostworld* (2001), *The Crow* (1994) and *The Craft* (1996), more often identifying with the freaks. I will always remember the famous line from *The Craft*, in which teen witch Nancy Downs, played by Fairuza Balk, replies to the bus driver who warns her to watch out for weirdos: 'We are the weirdos, Mister.' I felt seen.

Away from the big screen, I read bits of Baudelaire, Mary Shelley, H P Lovecraft and Edgar Allan Poe, and tried to make sense of the delirious ramblings of Aleister Crowley. To lull my adolescent angst, I listened to the dark symphonies of Siouxsie and the Banshees, The Sisters of Mercy, Bauhaus, The Cure and The Cramps. Meanwhile, I had posters of Winona Ryder, Rose McGowan and Angelina Jolie – in her vial-of-blood-wearing era – plastered to my walls. When I grew up I wanted to be just like them: gothic girls who revelled in after-dark mysteries and dressed in colours of the night. They were dangerous, they spoke up, and they refused to be defined by submissive femininity.

Art provided another form of refuge. I remember the first time I visited Tate Britain as a child and saw *Sleeping Venus* (1944) by the Belgian painter Paul Delvaux, and being completely enraptured. A subversion of the classical

3

sleeping Venus archetype, here was an image of a naked woman who had been ripped from the quiet domesticity of a bedroom and placed incongruously in a deserted town centre under the moonlit sky. A skeleton and a dressmaker's dummy watch over her in a play between life and death, the animate and inanimate, while background nudes thrash their hands around in anguish in this gothic fever dream.

At school, I would lose myself in art books about Gothic architecture and the 19th-century Gothic Revival. But it was the subversive work of German Surrealist Hans Bellmer which captivated me the most. Inspired by Jacques Offenbach's 1851 opera *The Tales of Hoffmann*, in which the hero falls in love with a mechanical doll, Bellmer spent the mid-30s building two life-size dolls out of wood, plaster and metal rods. Stylized in the form of young girls, with little white socks and Mary Jane shoes, Bellmer would place them in erotically charged scenarios and photograph their partially dismembered bodies, inviting the viewer of these hand-coloured images to engage in a voyeuristic game of fetishistic possibilities. Sure, it was dark, but it was also pretty mesmerizing.

While I got my teenage kicks through art, music, film and literature, it was through clothes and makeup that I was able to grapple with notions of identity. As I waged a silent war against the attrition of womanhood, my body became a battleground to be reclaimed. I filled my ears with piercings and never went anywhere without a velvet choker or spiked leather dog collar. Trawling through vintage shops on Portobello Road and flea markets on family holidays, I curated a uniform of black miniskirts and long black dresses which I wore with ripped tights, a hoodie and my trusty pair of Doc Marten boots, sometimes adding an ironic pop of lurid colour to throw people off the scent. Back then, I never considered beauty as a choice, but rather a necessary armour with which I could shield myself and my sadness from the world. This was at a point in my life when I didn't believe in makeup remover. The devil's juice, or so I thought. Instead, I would go to sleep each night with a fresh lick of mascara and another wring of kohl for that perfect 'slept-in' (read: punched-in-the-face) look. This routine would last until day five when either a stye would emerge or clumps of soot started to congeal, whereupon I'd have to take it all off and begrudgingly start again. My approach to hair was equally contrived. On the surface, my long locks looked haphazard and messy, qualities which belied careful consideration and artful skill. I would make two small plaits, one on each side above the ear, that I would tie together at the back, to create a cushion of volume at the crown, which over time (my record was two weeks) would mat together with grease to form a tangled web. Styled into a deep side parting, I used the bulk of torn-out front bits to obscure my left eye, like an eye patch, only crafted out of human hair. In short, I was a dark feral pixie in need of a good wash. But at least I felt protected.

During those early teenage years, I had a hard time negotiating my femininity and loathed my developing body, and it was through the language of goth that I was able to come to terms with both. It's been that way ever since; at every important crossroad – from coming of (r)age to becoming an adult, through falling in and out of love, navigating the workplace, marriage, motherhood, and beyond – the gothic vernacular has been there to shepherd me throughout, and will no doubt see me through until the end. I owe a lot to goth, which is why I want to champion its ghoulish mores so that it might inspire, or at least comfort, others in the way it has done for me. But before we get on to that, we must go back to the very beginning, to when time's dead flowers first stood in deathly bloom.

Chapter II:
A brief history of goth

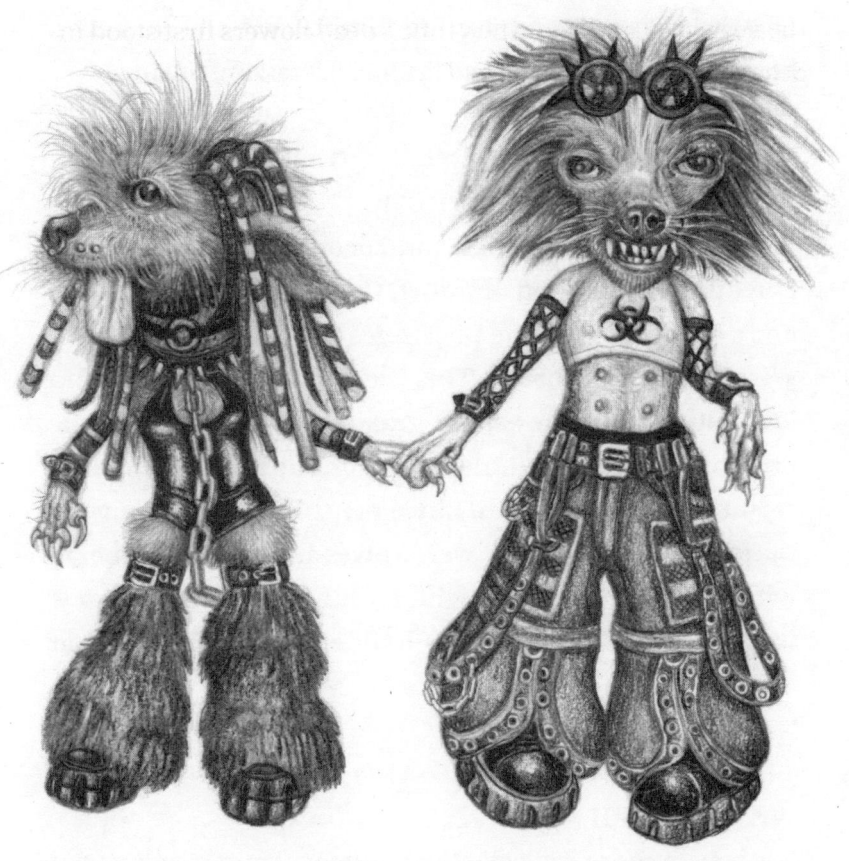

Since the sacking of Rome in AD 419 at the hands of the barbaric Visigoths, the term 'goth' has been encoded with ideas of death, destruction and decay. As every age brings about fresh horrors and a culture of darkness that springs up around it as a result, we may refer to this as the culture of goth. One that spans art, architecture, film, folklore and fairy tales; literature, poetry, music and fashion. Herewith: a primer.

THE DARK AGES: FUNGUS, GARGOYLES AND THE POINTED ARCH

A period defined by social and economic strife, the rise of feudalism, religious conflict, the spread of superstition and a deadly plague, the Dark Ages (the clue is in the name) were no laughing matter. This was echoed in both high and low culture, from the heaven-grazing, pointed arches of the great big Gothic cathedrals that sprung up across Europe – a result of technological advancements in construction – to the folky tales of witches, werewolves and the undead being whispered under candlelight. It didn't help that everyone was off their nut on ergot, a hallucinogenic fungus that affected the rye crops.

THE 16TH CENTURY: ROMEO MONTAGUE WAS A GOTH

With even more ecclesiastical upheaval and murmurs of geopolitical wars, writers like William Shakespeare and Christopher Marlowe started to embrace the cultural malady with sonnets about ghosts, melancholy and the macabre. Take Hamlet's famous soliloquy, for example, in which he ponders the possibility of death as being the only way to bring peace to his plight:

> To die, to sleep
> No more; and by a sleep, to say we end
> The heart-ache, and the thousand natural shocks
> That Flesh is heir to? 'Tis a consummation
> Devoutly to be wish'd.

It's the same with ol' Romeo 'I am fortune's fool' Montague. Fast-forward four or so centuries, and you know he'd be dousing himself in hairspray and hitting up the Batcave nightclub looking for bad romance.

THE 17TH CENTURY: POST TENEBRAS LUX

After the darkness comes the light. Without making too broad a statement, this was a pretty jammy period, defined by science, technology and rational thought. These were the halcyon days of Enlightenment, the Sun King and Newton's apple. As a result, across Europe the culture was grand, celebratory and Baroque – and therefore scant on gothic action.

THE 18TH CENTURY: STRAWBERRY HILL HORROR

Darkness returns. The cogs of the Industrial Age began turning and Europe was plagued by fear of what the dawn of the machine would mean for man, not to mention being ravaged by violent revolutions and very rampant disease. Against this backdrop of doom and disorder, the politician

Horace Walpole took to his sprawling gothic mansion, Strawberry Hill, and penned the 1764 novella *The Castle of Otranto*, a tale about hidden identities and supernatural forces, which would go on to inspire a full-blown Gothic Revival and spawn a new genre of horror. Not long after, the period's answer to Jilly Cooper, Ann Radcliffe, began writing her spooky chick-lit masterpiece *The Italian* (1796). Less preoccupied with graphic horror than she was with romance, the sublime and suspense, Radcliffe's writings still carry influence among *The Twilight Saga* tweekers today.

THE 19ᵀᴴ CENTURY: MOURNING GLORY

It was over a long, unnaturally gloomy Swiss weekend in June 1816, that the lothario Lord George Gordon Byron ('mad, bad, and dangerous to know', as his ex once described him) challenged his guests to a ghost-story writing competition, out of which came Mary Shelley's frenzied *Frankenstein, Or The Modern Prometheus* (1818) and John Polidori's *The Vampyre* (1819). Shortly afterwards the Irish author Bram Stoker published his own dystopian tale about a blood-drinking count.

Back in England, working conditions were squalid and mortality rates sky high, particularly among infants. A morbid fascination with the grotesque was considered *de rigueur*, particularly during the latter half of the period, when grief and mourning seemed to sum up the cultural mood. This was articulated through the rise of death masks, death portraits, lavish funerals and elaborate grave monuments, and communicated sartorially through a national dress code of black. Men accessorized with black armbands while women wore jewellery made of jet and trinkets that had belonged to loved ones, filled with locks of the deceased's hair – a movement that was inspired by Queen Victoria herself. Having lost her husband Albert after 21 years of marriage, aged just 38, she never let a scrap of colour touch her regal flesh again and built a giant, gilded, gothic monument to her prince in Hyde Park.

Nightmarish images continued to pervade culture in all its forms. Not just in England, but in Paris, too, where the poet Charles Baudelaire was putting pen to parchment about a putrefying corpse in his seminal *Les Fleurs Du Mal* (1857), the tropes of which were echoed more than a century later in many post-punk and goth lyrics, from Bauhaus and Siouxsie Sioux to Nick Cave and The Doors. Looking for someone to share his anguish with, it was Baudelaire who translated the tormented musings of American poet Edgar Allan Poe into French, another much-referenced figure within goth subculture.

THE 20TH CENTURY: A GOTHIC EXPLOSION

Welcome to a brave new world: a dynamic time that saw the birth of modern art, jazz and the sexually empowered flapper amid the rise of fascism and two grisly world wars. Much of the culture that defined the first half of the 20th century looked to make sense of these turbulent times through even darker material. Influenced by Poe, occultist writers H P Lovecraft and Aleister Crowley wrote sinisterly about sex and dark magic – themes that would later possess the lyrics of everyone from David Bowie to gothic rock band Fields of the Nephilim.

Bela Lugosi and the Scream Queens

In cinema, the genre of horror was beginning to take shape, thanks to French director Georges Méliès, who opened up the artistic possibilities of the medium with a host of spooky special effects. Among the more notable films of the period, there were *Les Vampires* (1915), *The Cabinet of Dr. Caligari* (1920), *Nosferatu* (1922), *Dracula* (1931) and *Frankenstein* (1931), which made a star out of genre actor Bela Lugosi. Years later, a still from *The Cabinet of Dr. Caligari* would appear on the back cover of Bauhaus's gothic anthem 'Bela Lugosi's Dead' (1982).

The dawn of gothic cinema also gave rise to a new female archetype: the femme fatale. Embodied both on and off screen by silent movie stars Theda Bara, Pola Negri, Nita Naldi and Jeanne Roques (also known as Musidora), these scream queens of early 20th-century cinema have a lot to answer for in terms of the traditional goth aesthetic; most of them were celebrated as much for their dark and decadent *maquillage* as for the vampy characters they inhabited.

Prompted by the discovery of Tutankhamun's tomb and all its treasures in 1922, Egypt-mania swept through Europe and America, inspiring cinema's leading ladies to cultivate mysterious off-screen personas to maximize their star potential. They dressed in arcane and 'exotic' costumes, with Cleopatra-style eye makeup consisting of thick kohl lines, geometric wings, painted brows and lashings of mascara. To stand out on black and white film, the look was finished off with blood-red lips (although this translated as black on screen) and thick matte foundation.

The Price Is Right vs Under The Hammer

Whereas the 30s had Bela Lugosi, the 50s had Vincent Price, the American actor known affectionately as the 'King of Horror', whose performances in *House of Wax* (1953) and *The Fly* (1958) came to define an entire genre of film, while *Cry of the Banshee* (1970) went on to inspire the name of one very famous goth band. Even more influential was sultry screen siren Maila Nurmi, otherwise known by her stage name, Vampira. With her jet-black hair, pallid skin and blood-red lips, together with her long black gown with its cinched-in waist and tentacle-like sleeves, she was the ultimate goth prototype. Even more titillating entertainment came courtesy of fetish superstar and 1955 *Playboy* centrefold Bettie Page, whose seamed stockings and signature curl-ironed fringe, dubbed the 'Bettie bangs', have gone on to influence a whole subset of rockabilly goths today.

In England, Hammer Film Productions, founded originally in 1934, was giving Hollywood and Price a run for their money, with a series of gory and darkly erotic films like *The Curse of Frankenstein* (1957) and *Dracula* (1958).

The American Nightmare

With rock and roll in full swing, the 60s saw the dawn of a darker and druggier scene. Drawing on the feverish sounds of Screamin' Jay Hawkins and his bewitching anthem, 'I Put A Spell On You' (1956), came British artists like the Undertakers and Screaming Lord Sutch. Across the pond, something else was brewing. Enter The Velvet Underground, whose sombre lyrics and sultry aesthetic coincided with teens becoming increasingly disillusioned – which were themselves only a recent invention. The term 'teenager' came into popular parlance only in the late 40s, as the demographic it referred to began to claw some semblance of independence away from the watchful eyes of their parents, which the mass availability of cars greatly contributed to. No longer perceived as children or mini-adults, grumpy teens became a movement in their own right, one that began to demand its own culture, tastes and values.

Unlike post-war Britain, which was defined by misery and austerity, post-war America was experiencing an economic boom. Everything was space agey and optimistic, as Americans celebrated the boundless possibilities of the future, quite literally launching themselves to the moon. The period also saw the rise of the American Dream, with white picket fences and shiny happy housewives. In reaction to this came sardonic shows like *The Munsters* (1964–6), *The Addams Family* (1964–6) and *Dark Shadows* (1966–71), along with horror hostess and campy goth pin-up Cassandra Peterson, *aka* Elvira.

Sex and Violence

By the early 70s, the world of entertainment had exploded into a multi-billion-pound industry, and cultural references to sex, violence and excess became more and more extreme. At one end, you had the futuristic drag and sexual fluidity of glam rock, brought to life via *The Rocky Horror Picture Show* (1975), the genre-defying musical about a 'sweet transvestite from transexual Transylvania' while, at the other end of the spectrum, the extreme pornographic imagery, bondage clothing and reappropriated Nazi ephemera of punk and violent films like *A Clockwork Orange* (1971) caused unease. Somewhere in the middle was the American musician Alice Cooper, whose turbocharged stage presence would go on to help define the goth subculture as we know it.

In Goth We Trust

It was out of punk and glam rock's hinterland and the maudlin musings of Joy Division, that ominously named bands like Alien Sex Fiend, Sex Gang Children, Southern Death Cult and The Sisters of Mercy began to emerge. Elsewhere, steeped in the tropes of gothic art and literature, Bauhaus gave us synth-driven, saturnine songs about bats, Bela Lugosi and the undead, brought to life with funereal sounds and eerie vocals; Siouxsie Sioux and the Banshees gave us shrill cries and sinister guitar strings; while angst-ridden lyrics came courtesy of The Cure. Forged in the UK's hellish fires of 1979, after a string of strikes, national acts of violence and the ascent of the much-maligned Margaret Thatcher, it was the music the world deserved.

By 1982, many goth bands had begun to play together, often congregating at London's hallowed underground nightclub the Batcave, where inky fiends came to lose themselves in gothic abandon. The nightclub was a key feature of the subculture, a stage upon which a rich tapestry of sartorial codes would play out. In Leeds there was Phono, Planet X in Liverpool, the Berlin Club in Manchester and the Tin Can in Birmingham. Even beyond England, nocturnal temples were sprouting up all over the world, as safe havens where goths could be themselves and find a sense of belonging in an increasingly frightening world.

Much has been written about goth and its parameters. While there has never been any fixed treaty or manifesto demarcating what it means (it wasn't given a name until the movement was well underway, while most of its prominent hellraisers would deny even being involved), it may be loosely articulated as a subterranean music and style scene unified by an aesthetic of darkness.

While punk was about the working-class hero rioting against the oppression of the government and the tyranny of the upper class, goth was romantic, and steeped in somewhat dandy ideals in its referencing of gothic art, architecture, film and literature. That said, goth owes much of its individualism and DIY, fetishistic aesthetic to the punk movement, in particular the provocative wares of Malcolm McLaren and Vivienne Westwood, whose iconic Kings Road shop, SEX, sold everything from gimp masks to ripped T-shirts emblazoned with swastikas, safety pins, images of mass murderers and pornographic stills.

But goth also took much of its visual lexicon from glam rock: the glittery romance and otherworldly androgyny of Marc Bolan and David Bowie, which it coupled with the camp theatrics of the New Romantics, with their swashbuckling frills and ostentatious ruffles.

Like all post-war subcultures, modern-day goth was born out of a desire to buck the system, and the most obvious way to do that was with your appearance, the aim being to shock and confront. Taking their cues from their favourite band members, women wore elements of historical costume such as big skirts, bodices and corsets, rendered in rich materials such as velvet, satin or lace, which they subverted with notes of PVC, latex and dominatrix leather. Men were equally flamboyant and performative, blurring the boundaries of gender with their piercings, nail polish, makeup and frilly romantic shirts, worn incongruously with combat boots and distressed leather jackets.

It was the same for beauty; the twin influences of punk and glam rock could be found in the goth's carefully curated palette of blacks (punk) and vivid blues, fiery reds and electric purples (glam), most of which were used around the eye area to menacing effect. Lips were smeared with crimson, blackcurrant or jet, and skin was rendered deathly thanks to chalky foundation and deep purple blusher under the cheekbones to mimic the sinister contours of those beyond the grave. Meanwhile, hair was styled into towering proportions, sprayed into stiff spikes, coiffed into crimped crow's nests and backcombed to oblivion, sometimes even shaved into 'deathhawks'. Black was the dominant colour, but acid tones, livid reds and bruised purples were also popular choices – anything that looked noxious and unnatural. Multiple piercings were another trope borrowed from punks, with goths often wearing chains in their noses that extended across to their ears. You know, the usual teenage stuff.

Red Velvet Lines the Black Box
By the time the 90s rolled around, most post-war subcultures had disbanded. Although it was a global movement, goth music, which had begun to embrace diverging industrial and EBM sounds, was beginning to fade away from mainstream

radio, TV and press coverage. But the spirit of goth rattled on in fringe fan zines, newsletters, alternative club nights and niche festivals such as the now biannual Whitby Gothic Weekend, and later via internet forums, giving the movement a newfound sense of mystery and exclusivity that most scene veterans revelled in.

Style began to evolve, too. Coinciding with the birth of rave culture and its crossover with the Japanese Lolita scene, goths started somewhat ironically to embrace pops of lurid colour, in particular red, pink and purple, which they juxtaposed with subverted childhood imagery and more obvious symbols of horror like vampire fangs and spooky contact lenses.

Thanks to their rejection of accepted cultural norms and their general aesthetic of doom and gloom, goths were widely viewed with suspicion, derision and ridicule, as strange misfits who lurked in the shadows, often represented in popular culture (mostly teen movies) as being the antithesis of cool, and even, in the wider media, as being falsely associated with acts of violence. Take the 1999 Columbine High School massacre, for example, which was unfairly blamed on controversial iconoclast Marilyn Manson, who had become something of a saviour for disenfranchised youths, and whose disturbing lyrics were claimed by the media to have incited the Columbine High School shooters to violence. Goth scene snobbery, however, would have you believe that Manson was never a true goth in the first place, despite his monstrous appearance and morbid exhibitionism. And perhaps, given the recent accusations of sexual assault against him, goths are right to reject him.

At the same time, wider culture hadn't quite satiated its appetite for the macabre, which probably had something to do with the post-Reagan recession, and the American real estate market crash. Amid a backdrop of national mourning, goth found a home on the big and small screen, most notably in the work of Tim Burton, in particular *Edward Scissorhands* (1990), whose titular character, played by Johnny Depp, bears a striking resemblance to The Cure's Robert Smith. There was also *The Addams Family* (1991), *Bram Stoker's Dracula* (1992), *The Crow* (1994), *Interview with the Vampire* (1994) and *The Craft* (1996). Meanwhile, on TV, shows like *Buffy the Vampire Slayer* (1997–2003) were finding keen audiences among disgruntled teens as they tried to make sense of a cruel world.

THE 21ST CENTURY: GRAVE TIMES

At the start of the 21st century, things were still bubbling away, but only if you knew where to look for them. The *Emily the Strange* and *Twilight* franchises were among the few mainstream conduits for the scene's newer, younger audiences. By this point, the style had atomized into a series of subgenres: you had the future-facing cybergoths who loved raving, science fiction and listening to techno. Taking their sartorial cues from films like *Blade Runner* (1982) and *The Matrix* (1999), cybergoths were recognizable for their black leather trench coats, goggles or dark shades and oversized footwear, which they wore with phosphorescent rave markings and humanoid elements like rubber tubing, fibre optics and even LEDs in their hair.

Equally preoccupied with technology, but through the lens of the past, the steampunk movement fused futuristic dressing with vintage Victoriana, which manifested sartorially in the marriage of humanoid gadgets with corsets, bodices and bustles for women and frock coats, top hats and canes for men. This affection for historical Victorian dress was shared by trad goths and vampire worshippers alike.

But it wasn't all cyborgs and high-tech futurism. In fact, there was one subset of goth that took its cues from the natural world and pre-Christian iconography. Spearheaded by bands such as All About Eve and Inkubus Sukkubus, this movement focused more on Wiccan magic than it did on horror, looking to ritualistic Pagan, often Celtic, dress to inform their style lexicon. It's giving sage-burning Sanderson sisters with their medieval tunics and hippy festival flower wreaths. Most likely to be spotted at the Stone Circle in Glastonbury discussing their plans for the next equinox.

Elsewhere, the gothabilly scene paid homage to 50s pinups like Bettie Page, brought back to life via pencil skirts, fishnet tights, beehives and exaggerated wings. Meanwhile, steeped in the cloying candy colours of gothic Lolitas, perky goths were defined by their cutesy brand of Halloween theatrics. Cue: witchy stockings and frilly miniskirts, backpacks emblazoned with cobweb designs and T-shirts embroidered with sparkly skulls.

Though clearly defined within the parameters of their scenes, these subcultures existed well beyond the masses, banished to the cultural badlands, where they remained until goth's current-day resurrection.

Chapter III:
Goth apocalypse now

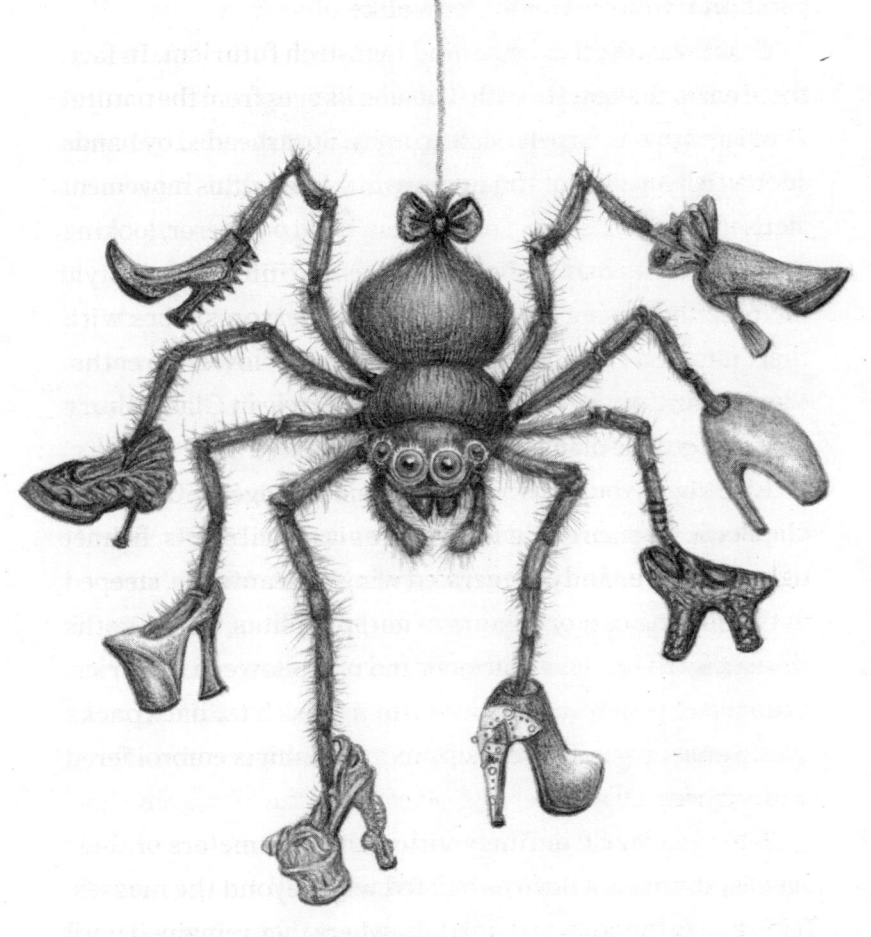

As we have seen, goth has meant different things to different people, from a violent Germanic tribe who sacked the great city of Rome to a historic style of art, architecture and literature, and latterly a specific style and musical subculture defined by its eldritch aesthetic. As well as obvious connotations of darkness, there is one thing that unites all of the above, and that is the notion of the outsider/disruptor/rebel, which is what goth has largely come to signify today – someone who identifies outside of the norm and who is drawn towards dark matter.

Back in the 80s, to be a goth meant to adhere to a set of shared, albeit unspoken, rules. But in today's post-subcultural world, to be a goth you no longer need to listen only to goth music, hang out only in goth clubs or dress strictly in black. Instead, goth is all around us, and you can dip in and out of the culture as you please. It's about being goth-coded. Indeed, thanks to modern sorcery, we can now move from one genre of music to another with a swipe of a button. It's the same for sartorial choices; one day you might be wearing a 40s tea dress and the next, a tracksuit from cult streetwear brand Palace, or possibly even layering them together in some weird anachronistic mash-up. Today, you can be everything, everywhere, all at once. Instead of subcultures, we now have 'cores': detached from any musical scene, these are stylized aesthetics that are born on TikTok and spill out into real life. There's cottagecore, an aesthetic devoted to romanticized notions of rural living; fairycore, which deals in notions of fantasy and magic; and goblincore, which embraces the more sinister side of nature.

Dark times produce dark culture and, as I think we can all agree, right now we're in a pretty dark place. From the death knells of looming world wars and increased religious unrest to the doomsday calls of Extinction Rebellion, not to mention the scars of a global pandemic that forced us to confront the fragility of our mortal coil, we are living in an unprecedented state of malaise and malcontent. Not to mention rising living costs, post-Brexit fallout in the UK, crippling inflation, a mental health crisis and a general housing shortage. Amid these waking nightmares, the solace of goth looms to soothe our morbid anxieties, infecting pop culture at every orifice. On top of this, thanks to the immediacy of social media and the cultural impetus of being permanently hooked up to our smartphones, culture – whether that's art, fashion, film, beauty, music or interiors – has never been more readily available to us, allowing things that once lurked in the shadows to be brought into the light. That's not to say goth has lost any of its subversive edge – far from it – rather, that this edge has found a wider audience. As we move through the roaring 2020s, the bats have once again left the bell tower and the victims have been bled. Let's take a closer look.

THE WITCH'S WARDROBE

From the runway and the red carpet to the internet highways via the street, gothic fashion is having a revival. Take the autumn/winter 2023 catwalk shows: at Balenciaga, a funeral procession of black-clad models came marching down the runway dressed in a series of oversized tailoring looks. There were notes of health goth, too (the 2014 viral lifestyle trend which fused fitness and biotech with a shadowy sensibility), with models wearing sporty Lycra bodies and angular velour tracksuits teamed with futuristic black sunglasses. Hair was gelled down reminiscent of 90s-style ravers, and accompanied by the odd deep berry lip.

Meanwhile, fashion's dark overlord and health goth daddy, the American designer Rick Owens, sent monstrous figures down his runway in black contact lenses and enormous platform boots. Proportions were exaggerated; black bulbous forms devoured models' torsos while high, angular collars crept out of caviar-hued leather coats.

At Erdem, designer Erdem Moralıoğʻlu looked to Victorian erotica and Charlotte Perkins Gilman's 1892 horror novella *The Yellow Wallpaper*, about a woman suffering from hysteria, to inform his sombre collection of tailored coats and dramatic taffeta skirts. There were also gothic moments at Christian Dior, Simone Rocha, Versace and Alexander McQueen, and the usual assault of black at Junya Watanabe and Yohji Yamamoto.

It's no coincidence that some of the biggest models of the moment are rooted in the gothic aesthetic, whether that's Vittoria Ceretti, Mariacarla Boscono or Amelia Gray. Even those shadowy musicians Arca, FKA twigs and Ethel Cain have taken to the catwalk and fronted recent campaigns. Elsewhere, mistress of darkness – and Rick Owens's wife – Michèle Lamy, has had more glossy-magazine covers in the last few years than you can shake an ornate claw-topped cane at. Meanwhile, Spanish actress and Pedro Almodóvar's dark muse, Rossy de Palma, was tapped to front Saint Laurent's autumn/winter 2023 campaign.

Away from high fashion, streetwear brands are also dabbling in the dark arts. Nike's recent collaboration with cult designer Yoon Ahn was brought to life in a short film inspired by 90s witch-flick *The Craft*, starring Amelia Gray-doppelganger Gabbriette Bechtel and shaven-browed beauty Josephine Lee, *aka* Princess Gollum, in which a group of ghoulish schoolgirls begin to embrace their supernatural powers. Designer Marc Jacobs tapped spooky songstress Doja Cat to star in a campaign for his youth-focused sub-line Heaven, as well as releasing a *Donnie Darko*-inspired drop with a series of dark and twisted visuals shot by the film's director, Richard Kelly.

As with the proliferation of any popular trend, the Kardashians have a lot to answer for. Teaming up with Italian fashion house Dolce & Gabbana on her 2022 wedding to punk rocker Travis Barker, Kourtney Kardashian and her koven of raven-haired sisters were seen dripping in lace and crucifixes like noir femmes fatales, and the bride was even pictured in a black veil in the days preceding. It heralded a darker direction for reality TV's favourite family, one that is still very much felt today in Kim Kardashian's black widow wardrobe. Even younger sister Kylie Jenner has gone over to the dark side with her vampirina looks, courtesy of deliciously gothic designer Dilara Findikoglu.

Away from the red carpet, the #goth and #gothgirl aesthetic are racking up 18.5 and 5.6 billion hits respectively on TikTok since inception, where users go to wallow in the abyss and share their sultry, sullen looks. Meanwhile, on Instagram, Berlin-based fashion editor Brenda Weischer, otherwise known as Brenda Hashtag, has been carving out her own minimalist take on the goth aesthetic, relying heavily on Rick Owens pieces and second-hand Ann Demeulemeester, which she mixes up with monochromatic images of modern art and mid-century furniture. In fact, Instagram has become an integral space through which contemporary articulations of goth (which is to say a much more normcore manifestation of the movement) are given form. For example, the British stylist and creative director Betsy Johnson's profile typically comprises a patchwork of Balenciaga-clad models, blurry images of black leather accessories and close-up shots of incongruous items, such as a pair of feet with painted black nails, her face bloody from a nosebleed, some bondage gear and a still from some obscure horror movie.

DISCO INFERNO

There's been a saturnine shift in music, too. Billie Eilish's spiked dog collars and lobotomized stare, coupled with her morose meditations on the human condition, make her the ultimate goth icon. Equally miserable are the SoundCloud rappers, those disenfranchised teens with dyed hair and face tattoos, who rap nihilistically about Xanax addiction and broken America, and the lugubrious lyrics of Yung Lean and his Swedish Sad Boys. Covered in tattoos, they bridge the style gap between goth and football casual, with their ironic polo shirts and spooky harlequin-inspired face paint. Bladee, Varg2™, Ecco2K and the rest of the Drain Gang are another Swedish export dealing in notions of the macabre with their chilling lyrics and sinister heavy metal looks.

Of course, one can't talk about goth without mentioning British artist FKA twigs, who combines haunting vocals with nightmarish imagery and a macabre beauty aesthetic that has seen her embrace monstrous contact lenses and extraterrestrial markings. Or the American rapper 070 Shake, otherwise known as Danielle Balbuena, who makes maudlin music about microdosing and astrology, is covered in tattoos and rarely strays from her strict wardrobe of black. That she rose to fame after her lyrics 'I put my hand on the stove, to see if I still bleed / And nothing hurts anymore, I feel kinda free' in Kanye West's 'Ghost Town' (2018) went viral is a testament to our current morbid climate.

Now more than ever, music has become as much of a visual medium as it is an auditory one, with music videos allowing artists to create parallel universes featuring all kinds of horrors and disturbing vignettes. Take experimental artist Yves Tumor, whose video for 'God Is a Circle' (2023) saw him metamorphose into a Mephistophelian creature dug up from the grave. Or American rapper Rico Nasty, whose ghoulish brand of glam saw her shapeshift into a host of surreal characters in the video for 'Own It' (2020), which featured severed dolls, a spiked gimp mask, shrimp heads and a distorted mermaid tail with finger-like fins. Equally dystopian is the dreamscape weaved by Venezuelan artist Arca in the video for 'Prada/Rakata' (2021), influenced by the Swiss biomechanical artist H R Giger and featuring alien-like figures, two-headed skeletons and the singer reimagined as a hybrid bat.

It's not just happening on the fringes. To accompany her haunting track 'Vampire' (2023), teen pop sensation Olivia

Rodrigo tapped photographer Petra Collins to direct a cloying fever-dream of a video inspired by 50s horror movies. Meanwhile, the self-described 'bad lil' bitch' Doja Cat has been petrifying the masses with her latest cycle of music videos, replete with grim reapers, horned creatures and apocalyptic disasters.

On top of that, 2023 saw the unexplained re-emergence of goth icon Siouxsie Sioux after a decade-long hiatus. Like a phoenix rising from the ashes of the 80s, she spent the summer headlining festivals and propping up stages across Britain, bewitching her black-clad audiences with her intoxicating magic. In the same year, The Sisters of Mercy stormed America, The Damned teased a comeback, Nick Cave returned to the studio and whispers of a new album from The Cure grew louder.

IDLE HANDS

Goth has cast its shadow over art, too. German artist Anne Imhof's 2022 *Avatar II* exhibition at Sprüth Magers' London outpost is a testament to that: from her deserted locker-room installation to her scratched-out aluminium panels, Imhof's dystopian vision of the world summed up the cultural mood. Then there's American artist Tiona Nekkia McClodden, whose subversive work about race, gender, sexuality and the spiritual world was the subject of not one but three exhibitions in 2022 alone. At MoMA, she showed a large video installation which drew on the rhetoric of BDSM and featured the artist hanging upside down while reciting a piece by the late poet Brad Johnson, while in *Mask/Conceal/Carry*, her exhibition at

David Zwirner gallery, she explored the practice of shooting a gun as a meditation on trauma and self-protection.

2023 was equally ripe with gothic art happenings. Sadie Coles gallery staged *Hardcore*, a group exhibition chronicling the agony and ecstasy of the human condition, featuring violent and sexually charged works from Cindy Sherman, Bruce LaBruce, King Cobra (*aka* Doreen Lynette Garner) and Tayeba Begum Lipi, among others. Elsewhere, American artist Lizzi Bougatsos contemplated bodily fragility in a solo show at TRAMPS gallery in New York. A series of installations comprising used bandages from when she accidentally caught on fire during a 2001 performance, *Idolize the Burn: An Ode to Performance* was a meditation on pain and resilience.

DAWN OF THE SLASHERS

Pre-empted by the *American Horror Story* (2011–) television show franchise, that pop cultural behemoth that has featured everyone from Cara Delevingne and Naomi Campbell to Kim Kardashian and Lady Gaga, recent times have seen a boom in goths on film. From Ti West's harrowing slasher trilogy *X* (2022), which follows the life of a bloodthirsty woman hungry for fame, to the *Scream* (2022) franchise reboot, what was once considered a niche, spine-tingling genre has now been accepted as part of the mainstream.

The dark lord of celluloid, Tim Burton, has also been working his black magic on the big and small screen with his upcoming *Beetlejuice* reboot and the smash-hit Netflix series *Wednesday* (2022). Starring Jenna Ortega, who is carving out a name for herself as horror's leading lady, the series follows the misadventures of Gomez and Morticia's angst-ridden daughter as she navigates the choppy waters of adolescence. Particularly poignant is a scene in which the apathetic teen, ethereally beautiful in a black organza creation, dances hypnotically to The Cramps' gothabilly song 'Goo Goo Muck', which later sparked a viral trend on TikTok.

So, what does all this mean? In short: the world has descended into madness. It's time to embrace the chaos.

Chapter IV:
Coming of age as a goth:
notes on style

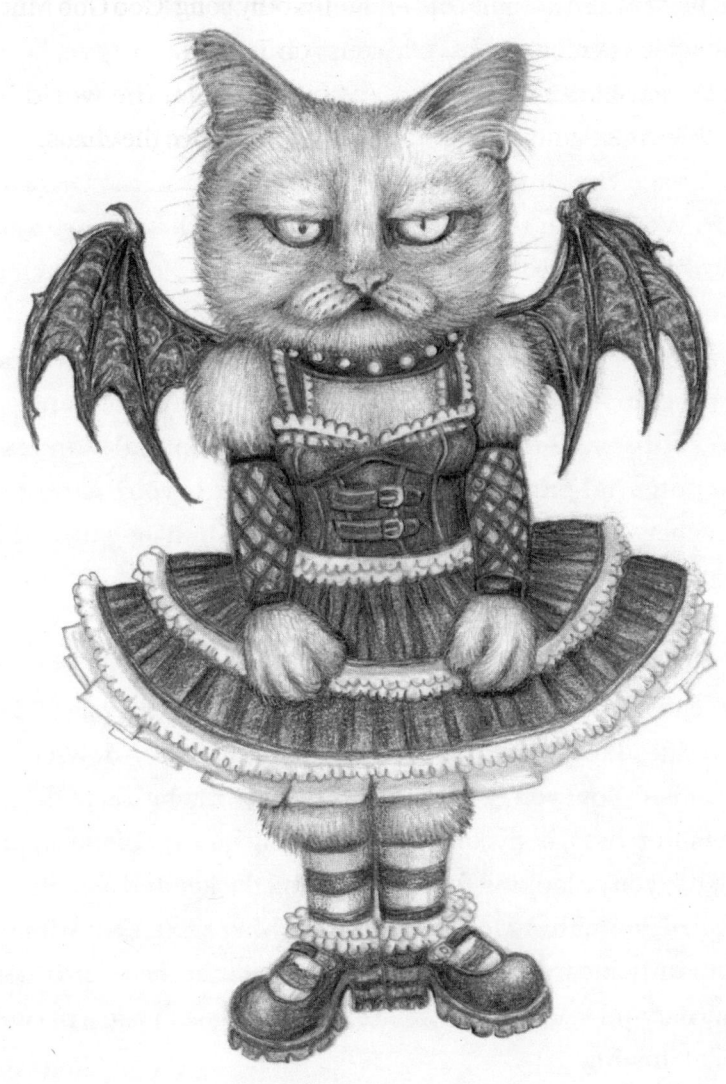

There's a famous scene in Sofia Coppola's seminal film *The Virgin Suicides* (1999) in which the youngest Lisbon daughter is lying in her hospital bed after her first suicide attempt. 'What are you doing here, honey?' her middle-aged male doctor says to her. 'You're not even old enough to know how bad life gets.' To which Cecilia replies: 'Obviously, Doctor, you've never been a 13-year-old girl.'

Being a teenager is the age where nothing fits. Caught between the shifting sands of childhood and the Grown-Up World, you're desperate to find out who you are and how to navigate this thing called life. A tangle of blistering hormones and strange new body parts, you're cripplingly uncomfortable in your own skin and afraid that everyone can see it. As you try to negotiate the dichotomies of wanting to conform to the peer pressure of school pals, appeal to potential paramours and rebel against your parents/teachers/the patriarchy – to look hot, cool and ugly, all at the same time – your body becomes a battleground and style your weapon of choice.

Of course, the easiest thing to do sartorially is to fade into the background and coast along as part of the pack ('On Wednesdays we wear pink'). But you know deep down that that isn't you; you're not quite like those other girls with the push-up bras, bodycon dresses and big bouncy blonde hair. What you're looking for is something darker and a bit more weird, something to soothe your aching anxieties. Which can only mean one thing: it's time to embrace your inner outlier and lean into the solace of goth. Welcome to a period of mourning.

Inspired by frontwomen Siouxsie Sioux, Christine Wade of Alien Sex Fiend and Patricia Morrison of The Sisters of Mercy and The Damned, in the 80s goths would spend hours dressing their bodies in a tableau of symbols, textures and objects that were thrifted, mail ordered or specially handmade. Although no goth wanted to look like another, there were obvious style codes: a DIY mix of historical costume and notes of BDSM. Fast-forward to today's post-subcultural landscape, however, and things are much more fluid.

Guiding someone through their style journey inevitably takes away some of the fun of figuring it all out for themselves; stylistic tribulations often end up being more rewarding than rarer triumphs. Because, ultimately, style is a maiden voyage of self-discovery. If the path is already determined, what is there to learn? That said, suggestions can be made, and should be. After all, these are trying times for the individual, what with all the algorithmic echo chambers ramming homogeneity down our throats. Luckily, with its rich visual history and cavernous references, goth is a treasure trove to be mined – you just need to know how to approach it without succumbing to pastiche. This comes down to inventiveness, finding the right pieces and assembling them in a way that feels contemporary and unique.

Where to start? At the mercy of your parents' purse strings and/or the spoils of a weekend job, here's where the young goth must get creative: customizing clothes, pillaging family wardrobes (Mum, Dad, older siblings), traversing charity shops, markets, and thrift stores, and mining eBay,

Vinted and Depop for lost gold. Blending high and low, vintage and modern, the key is to mix your second-hand garbs with expertly curated high-street fits, leaning into unusual juxtapositions and proportions, and not relying too much on one thing (unless we're talking about the colour black). What you're striving for is individuality, which comes from sourcing things from far and wide. Throw everything at the cave wall and see what sticks – old Army surplus boots, DIY ripped tights from John Lewis, a Y2K Blumarine slip dress from Depop, and a bashed-up leather jacket from Portobello Market. Then bring in other style codes, too, such as your Shox MR4 × Martine Rose Nike trainer-mules or classic Carhartt double-knee pants. To dress in a modern way today, it's all about an eclectic mix of things.

This approach will see you through university, art school, and the underpaid internship years when money is as tight as a corset, emotions run high and true independence remains just outside your claws. Bloated on poststructuralist discourse, Marxist theories and feminist ideologies, throughout these years of young adulthood you've never been more aware of the malleability of your identity. And it is through style that you can masterfully hone it. Where in your teens you might have shied away from the more extreme shock tactics of goth, what better way to round off these final coming-of-age moments than by relinquishing yourself to true gothic abandon? Here's where a bit of hardcore bondage gear comes in handy: a latex dress from some specialist fetish store teamed with an oversized stripey mohair jumper, some fishnets, brothel creepers and a spiked dog collar.

As you navigate the tectonic shifts of adolescence and the blur of hormones that comes with it, this can be one of the most excruciating times in your life. And doing it as someone who doesn't fit the prescribed mould, whether by design or default, is infinitely harder. But it can also be the most rewarding experience. Grappling with notions of independence for the first time, this is the period in which you start to develop your tastes, your tribe, your politics, what you stand for and what you stand against. It's ultimately the period in which you start to find yourself, or at least some semblance of self in an ever-shifting world. Among all this, finding your style might seem trivial, but in fact these are all pieces of the same puzzle, and what you sometimes can't put into words, you might well be able to articulate through the language of clothes – and this will put you in good stead for the hurdles that come ahead.

STYLE CHECKLIST: THE ESSENTIALS

The leather jacket

Popularized in the 50s by lean, mean on-screen bad boys Marlon Brando and James Dean in films like *The Wild One* (1953) and *Rebel Without a Cause* (1955), the leather jacket is a well-worn symbol of youthful dissidence, and practically every post-war subculture has enjoyed their own iteration of it. With its origins in military wear, from the 60s onwards, young women started to embrace it as a way to toughen up their image and in doing so stick two fingers up to the patriarchy. With its rich, subversive history, the leather jacket remains a potent semaphore of teen rebellion today. But it has to be black, and it has to be vintage. Whether it's an original, oversized 50s Harley-Davidson biker jacket in pristine condition or a second-hand, tailored trench coat, it needs to have some age to it. And you can find these in pretty much any vintage market or thrift shop, all over the world. Since it adds an element of harshness to your overall look, it's best worn with something soft or delicate underneath as a contrast, such as a silk slip dress or tulle underskirt, worn with a shrunken cardigan or oversized mohair jumper.

Tights

Before becoming a staple, the humble pantyhose was once viewed as a symbol of female liberation. Invented in 1959 to relieve women from the tyranny of the girdle-garter-stockings complex, it came of age during the great 60s Youthquake and became instant partner-in-crime with the equally insurgent miniskirt. By the 80s, however, it wasn't enough to just wear tights, you had to wear them ripped and laddered, held together with safety pins and paired with winklepickers or Doc Martens. Fast-forward to today and the irreverent attitude of a pair of ripped tights remains just as formidable.

Fishnets are another weapon in the young goth's artillery of style. Originally worn in stocking form, they've been peeking out of ever-rising hemlines since their late 19th-century inception. Revealing more flesh than they conceal, they are duplicitous by nature and have been enjoyed as an erotic tease as a result. Associated with fetishism and underground club culture in the post-war period, they took on even greater significance in the 70s and 80s when worn ripped by the likes of punk icon Nancy Spungen and Siouxsie Sioux, who later traded in her fishnet tights for entire fishnet bodysuits. Just as transgressive today, they're an essential item of clothing for any fledgling goth.

The Victoriana nod

With their fetishization of all things dark and grotesque and strict codes of appropriate mourning dress, the Victorians were a pivotal influence on gothic style in the 20th century, and many goths chose to recreate the era verbatim via head-to-toe period dressing. But where in the 80s and 90s, Victorian dress felt new and rebellious, unless you're at a cosplay convention, today it verges on pastiche. The trick, then, is to mix certain Victorian elements with more contemporary pieces. Try throwing a tape-lace capelet or beaded mourning mantle over your favourite band T-shirt and a pair of black leather hot pants; wear a black bodice as if it's a jacket, open over a long slip dress; or layer a tailored frock coat over a latex mini. What you want is a nod to the era without it being too referential.

The babydoll dress

Cutesy and illicit, Japan's gothic Lolita scene came of age in the early 90s. Although steeped in an aesthetic of childish innocence – think big bows, pretty frills, Victorian petticoats and quaint Rococo bonnets – its association with adult themes of death and sex add an element of the perverse. Inspiring the perky goth movement in the West, from the mid-90s onwards the strict goth colour palette of black gave way to sherbet hues and cutesy childlike ephemera as goths morphed into undead dolls. A key trope of this movement was the babydoll dress. With its dual nature of eroticism and infantilism, which only intensified after its collision with the 90s Riot Grrrl movement, today the babydoll dress remains a symbol of female sexuality and rebellion, and has inspired many modern designers – from Molly Goddard and Simone Rocha to Cecilie Bahnsen – as a result. To give it a contemporary twist, opt for an asymmetric silhouette and pair it with fishnets, combat boots, a dog collar and a leather trench.

Corsets, lingerie and bondage gear

Once viewed as a token of oppression, in the 70s – under the stewardship of Dame Vivienne Westwood – women began wearing corsets as a form of armour, with underwear as outerwear becoming a new expression of female power. There was also something romantic about the corset's rich history that appealed to goths' dandyist ideals. It was the same for other items of lingerie, such as bodices, garters, girdles, suspenders and stockings, all of which were imbued with an anarchic power when worn in a nightclub setting. This was particularly the case when mixed with fetish and bondage wear such as rubber harnesses, latex bodysuits and studded leather bras, which by the 80s and 90s had become uniform for goths and cybergoths alike. Ideal for any brooding teen looking to rage against the machine, underwear as outerwear is an integral component of the gothic look. Keep it modern by playing around with textures and silhouettes; pair your corsets with oversized tailoring and your leather harness with a Peter Pan-collar tea dress – a nod to the original weird sister, Wednesday Addams.

The mohair sweater

A staple of the punk, goth and later grunge aesthetic, the oversized mohair sweater and its cardigan cousin are two of counterculture's cosiest items. A fuzzy blur of shag and wool, they're the perfect foil to all that latex and leather and will lend an ironic softness to any young goth's look. Best worn with a cervix-skimming miniskirt, opting for one with stripes is a great way to introduce a splash of colour to your otherwise all-black image.

Boots

New Rocks, winklepickers, Doc Martens, military boots – whatever your style preference, no gothic wardrobe is complete without a pair of sturdy boots. With their origins in military wear, the combative connotations of this footwear staple have long been associated with anti-establishment style. Adopted by skinheads and punks in the 70s, Doc Martens became a crucial hallmark of female rebellion, one that would appeal to goths in the following decade. For those witchier wonders like Siouxsie Sioux, who erred more towards the feminine, pointed winklepickers provided the perfect alternative, while cybergoths and steampunks of the late 90s gravitated towards the towering proportions and industrial feel of New Rock platforms. Remaining a symbol of sedition today, boots will lend a gritty realism and gravitas to any look. Get authentic combat boots from military surplus stores around the world or head to the Dr Martens store in Camden Market for the OG goth experience.

Creepers

During the 50s, thick-ridged, crepe-soled shoes with suede or leather uppers became one of the key signifiers of a new youth scene known as the teddy boys. Originally worn by WWII soldiers as they traipsed through the deserts of North Africa, they were renamed 'brothel creepers' due to their association with certain Soho nightspots, as well as a specific shuffle movement that was taking over the dancefloor. Since then, creepers have been embraced by practically every underground scene from punks, goths and rockabillies to the emos and indie kids of the early 21st century, and play a defining role in shaping any counter-cultural wardrobe today. A softer alternative to the archetypal goth boot, wear them day or night with ripped stockings and a babydoll dress or a sharply tailored trouser suit.

Accessories

Victorian mourning jewellery is another essential trope of gothic style. Fashioned from jet or other dark materials, these trinkets often contained a lock of the deceased's hair and were adorned with *memento mori* emblems, including skulls, something that would later capture the imagination of our young goth in the post-war period. It was Dame Viv who brought bones into punk's style lexicon, attaching them to chains and putting them on T-shirts to spell out words like 'Rock' and 'Perv'. In the 80s, goths would string boiled animal bones onto necklaces along with voodoo bags, or fix them onto earlobes as a nod to the occult. Other popular motifs included crosses, crucifixes and ankhs (an ancient religious symbol) – always in silver, never in gold – which tapped into the gothic fascination with vampires, religion and the undead. These were stacked on fingers, worn on wrists and jangled around necks, while spiked or chained leather dog collars and studded leather belts tapped into the hardcore fetish scene.

A key signifier of goth style today, these accessories can be worn day and night, layered or worn alone. Again, look for contrasts: wear a dog collar with a 30s bias-cut dress or an ankh with a bashed-up leather biker jacket.

NOTES ON BEAUTY

As we have seen, navigating the trenches of adolescence is no mean feat. During this period, if your body is to become a battleground, and style your weapon of choice, then makeup becomes your warpaint. This is particularly true for the young goth. Indeed, while everyone else around you seemingly turns to makeup as a way to camouflage or prettify themselves, for the young goth it's more a vital tool for self-expression.

I became a teenager in the autumn of 2003 (three weeks shy of Halloween), at a time when the dominant beauty trend was to transform yourself into a piece of confection – and this was light years before Hailey Bieber and her glazed doughnut skin. From frosted eyelids to honeyed lips (courtesy of Lancôme's Juicy Tube revolution), high-shine textures, saccharine hues and copious amounts of shimmer were considered *de rigueur*. Another prominent trend was to obscure your lips with concealer so all you could see of the lower half of your face was just skin, chin and enamel. Concealer worn under the eyes was always two shades lighter than your actual skin tone, foundation was two shades darker, and no teen would be caught dead without Maybelline's Great Lash Volumizing and Thickening Mascara, easily identified by its watermelon-hued packaging. Meanwhile, hair was piled scruffily onto heads, styled with butterfly clips, and occasionally sprayed with glitter or combed through with coloured mascara, its condition damaged from years of flat iron and Sun-In abuse. And the pungent smell of teen spirit came mingled with Veet, Vera Wang's Princess perfume and the biscuity notes of fake tan.

These days beauty is much less prescriptive, which is how it should be, especially during the coming-of-age period. Where previously your beauty choices were reflective of your tribe, today they are an expression of individuality. In the last few years, the beauty industry has undergone a major makeover. Emerging makeup artists are breathing new life into heritage beauty lines and dismantling antiquated ideals in their wake; everyday disruptors are democratizing the space with their huge online followings and viral how-to tutorials, which cover everything from niche drag to red carpet glam; meanwhile, conversations around race, gender, diversity, body positivity and identity are finally coming to the fore. Which is why, when it comes to beauty, there are now infinitely more ways to present as goth today. It's about finding what works for you.

If goths of years past were motivated by thumbing their noses at the establishment, the more extreme iterations of the style today are about petrifying it to its core. Take Hannah Rose Dalton and Steven Raj Bhaskaran, the otherworldly duo behind art, music and design movement Fecal Matter, who are never seen without their signature alien corpse paint. Think shaved heads, bleeding orifices, dyed black sclerae (the white parts of the eye) and ghostly vein-streaked faces, with their limbs often sprouting demonic fleshy horns. It's their way of expressing themselves and pushing the boundaries of what beauty can be, an endeavour that has seen them embraced by some of the fashion industry's most renowned names, from Rick Owens to Balenciaga. Equally morbid is Aryuna Tardis, the Russian TikTok star and makeup artist who has been scaring the masses with her gory prosthetics and inspiring a legion of uncanny lookalikes as a result.

At the other end of the spooky spectrum, there's 'succubus chic'. Coined by *Dazed and Confused* magazine, the term describes a cleaner, more veristic interpretation of vamp. It's good girls gone goth. Currently sweeping runways, editorials, social media and the street, and epitomized by the likes of models Gabbriette Bechtel and Amelia Gray, and musicians Dove Cameron and Arca, it transforms its wearer into a dark temptress with bleached or pencil-thin brows, over-lined 90s style glossy lips, subtle feline flicks and pitch-black locks. It was precisely this ghoulish glam aesthetic that lay at the heart of makeup artist Isamaya Ffrench's inaugural collection for her eponymous brand, which was launched in 2022.

But not all gothic statements of beauty are rooted in glam or even horror, for that matter. Take Ethel Cain, the enchanting alter ego of singer-songwriter Hayden Anhedönia, whose makeup-free visage and unpolished hair, coupled with the intricate tattoos scattered across her body – the word 'please' written on her neck, the sleeve of crucifixes on her arm, and the names Ashmedai (the king of all demons) and Gabriel (the archangel) written in Hebrew on her forehead – lend an unexpected naturalism to her otherwise witchy demeanour and spooky brand of theatrics. It's a similar aesthetic adopted by rising model Hunter Pifer, whose striking features and raw beauty have seen her on the catwalk for brands including Prada, Marc Jacobs, Valentino and Balenciaga. In fact, many of Balenciaga's gothic muses are notable for their anti-glam aesthetic: just look at any of the brand's runway shows or campaigns. In a world of photoshopped perfection, of fillers and filters, this rejection of traditional ideals of glamour in favour of a much grungier approach is perhaps more radical than the more extreme iterations of goth.

Much like gothic style, today's gothic beauty choices should be determined by the individual. And these coming-of-age years provide the perfect opportunity in which to explore and experiment. So do just that: leaf through street-style books documenting subcultures of the 80s; go on

TikTok; stalk beauty disruptors; study the raw beauty that makeup artist Inge Grognard crafts for Balenciaga's runway shows; watch Theda Bara's hypnotic turn in *A Fool There Was* (1915); channel that teen angst through livid red hues; soothe your raging hormones with charcoal-ringed eyes; get something pierced; bleach or shave your brows; streak your hair with lurid green; wake up the next day and do something entirely different; let your hair and makeup say something about who you are and who you want to be. There's never been a better time for it.

BEAUTY CHECKLIST: THE ESSENTIALS

Black eyeliner

Women have been accentuating their eyes with black since ancient Egyptian times, when it was customary to line the eyes in kohl as a way of enlisting protection from the gods and fighting off bacterial infections. It wasn't until the 20s however, that women began to embrace the style in the West, with cinema's most transgressive and alluring stars harking back to Orientalist icons Queen Nefertiti and Cleopatra, as a result of the Egyptology mania that was sweeping Europe and America. Since then, exaggerated wings, jet-black waterlines and kohl-smudged lids have been associated with a kind of dark romanticism – one that was adopted by goths to menacing effect. The obligatory warpaint for any angst-ridden teen, whether liquid, pencil or a kajal stick, applied precisely or smeared on, black eyeliner is a cornerstone in any modern goth's makeup kit. To make the look feel modern, keep the eyes the main focus, leaving the skin clean and dewy, the brows tidy and brushed, and the lips neutral with a nude matte. Or throw caution to the wind and go full witch with matching liquorice lips.

Piercings

Historically viewed as an affront to the Judeo-Christian idea of the body being made perfect in God's image, it was the punks who brought piercings into youth culture's vernacular, inspiring goths to festoon their bodies with studs, spikes, skulls, bones and chains in the years since. Synonymous with teen rebellion today, getting something pierced is a rite of passage for any young goth – a way of literally taking ownership over your body, whether by drunkenly letting a mate puncture your ear at a party or getting your septum spiked by a professional.

Tattoos

Like piercings, tattoos are a key characteristic of the gothic aesthetic. Subversive in their perceived perversion of the unmodified body, they've long been associated with acts of transgression, compounded by their historical association with criminals. But they also have connotations of the occult, with body art playing a vital role in various spiritual practices from around the world, something that has always appealed to the gothic fascination with mystery and the macabre. Whether it's a tattoo of a bat skeleton, like the one sprawled across Doja Cat's back, or any of the *memento mori* symbols that adorn Ethel Cain's body, getting something inked can be an essential part of growing up – even if you come to regret it later.

Hair dye

Buying your first bottle of hair dye and standing over the bathroom sink as you attempt to drastically alter your image is a rite of passage. In the 80s, black was the dominant hair colour for brooding creatures of the night, but by the end of the decade and well into the 90s and noughties, radioactive hues and vivid shades of red, pink and purple were becoming more and more ubiquitous. Today, switching up your hair colour remains a prerequisite for any young goth navigating their kidulthood. So get yourself down to the hair salon and opt for flame-red hues like Aryuna Tardis or buy a bottle of Billie Eilish-inspired slime-green dye and do it yourself at home.

Bleached or shaved brows

These days, bleaching or shaving your brows is the most obvious way to pledge allegiance to all things counter-cultural. Currently dominating the runway, social media and the street, invisible arches allow their wearer to shapeshift into something amorphous and otherworldly, especially when paired with a shaved head and demonic contact lenses, as in the case of Fecal Matter. But it doesn't always have to be so extreme. Model Gabbriette Bechtel often teams barely-there brows with her signature soft vamp look, while makeup artist Isamaya Ffrench pairs them with high-shine textures for an industrial glam effect.

Spooky contact lenses

Drawing on the iconography of horror, spooky contact lenses are a well-worn trope within certain goth subgenres, particularly those of the 90s and early noughties. For his autumn/winter 1997 collection, master of fantasy and spectacle Thierry Mugler sent shockwaves through the fashion industry when he transformed supermodel Adriana Karembeu into a monstrous creature replete with supernatural yellow contact lenses that he heightened using lurid blue and green eyeshadow. It's no less subversive today, so if you really want to scare people, rock a pair of white contact lenses and go about your day.

Chapter V:
Gothic heroines, part I

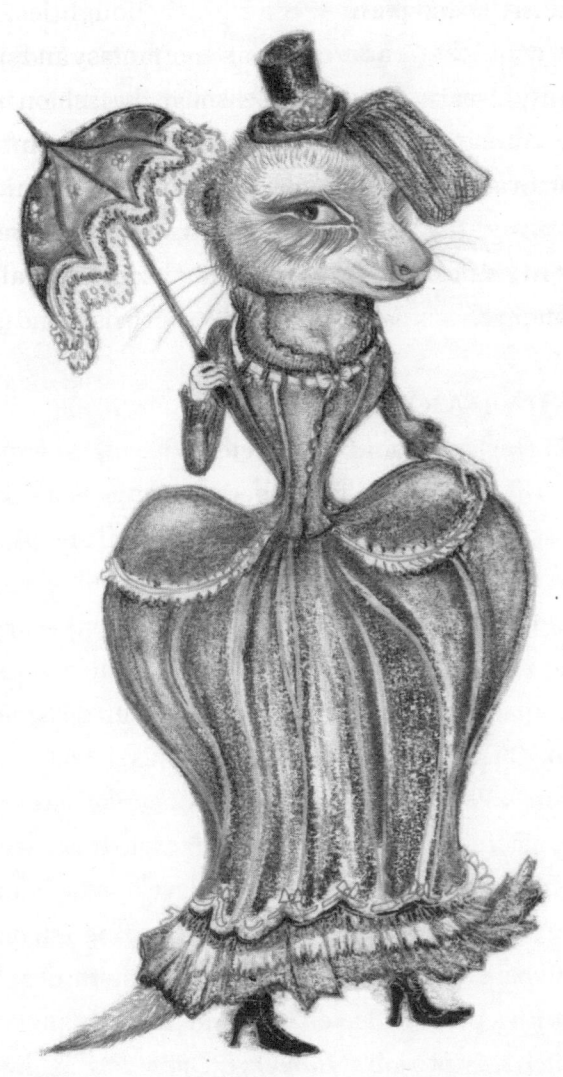

Distilling the world's greatest gothic icons into a 40-strong list was never going to be easy. Some choices will be obvious, their gothic credentials undeniable, while others may be more obscure, and some might not even define themselves as goths or gothic in the first place.

Nevertheless, each one has been chosen for their originality, creativity and fearlessness, not just in terms of their style but in the way they live their lives. From fictitious teen tearaways and historical screen sirens to distinguished novelists and tragic jilted brides, traversing time, space and reality, their contributions to the gothic canon are wide-ranging.

AMANDA HARLECH

Amanda Harlech would never refer to herself as a muse. It's too objectifying and old-fashioned, and suggests a passivity that grossly undermines the many hats (real and figurative) that she wears. Instead call her a consultant, conspirator or second-in-command, call her a stylist or style archivist, someone to bounce ideas off and drape haute couture on – qualities that have seen her work closely with designers John Galliano, Karl Lagerfeld and, most recently, Kim Jones.

Born in 1959, Harlech grew up in a bohemian house in north London, where she was encouraged to paint, draw, dance, play piano, play dress up, ride and act. She developed a flair for style in her early twenties, emerging from an English degree at Oxford (where she was drawn to the gothic literature of Henry James) with a punk-inflected look and partially shaved head, after which she got a job at *Harpers & Queen* as a fashion editor.

Forging a creative alliance with fashion's *enfant terrible* John Galliano, she would spend the next decade spinning rags into riches with him (what they lacked in money they made up for in creativity) both for his namesake label and during his stint at Givenchy.

When Galliano was offered a job at Dior, Harlech went to work with Karl Lagerfeld at Chanel and Fendi, where she traded in bias-cut chiffon dresses for haute couture tweed, until Lagerfeld died in 2019. Continuing her tenure at Fendi, she now works alongside the house's current creative director Kim Jones, to whom she lends her gothic sensibilities and knack for telling stories.

No one understands clothes quite like Harlech, which is just as evident in her style as it is in her work with her chosen designers. Steeped in the language of goth, she mixes high and low, vintage and contemporary, always dialling up the drama with some kind of theatrical accessory, whether it's a top hat and funereal veil, a pair of tulle opera gloves or some exotic plumes. That said, she looks just as good in a pair of jodhpurs and marigolds as she does on the red carpet: something we can all aspire to.

ANNE IMHOF

Fraught, fragile and foreboding, Anne Imhof makes messed-up art for our messed-up world. Her first-ever performance piece was staged back when she was working as a bouncer for a local nightclub in Frankfurt. Set in a bar in the red-light district, the piece was conceived as a one-night-only boxing match at which boxers were invited to fight for as long as a band was playing, while the band were instructed to play for as long as the boxers were fighting. Chaos ensued.

In 2017, Imhof represented Germany at the Venice Biennale and transformed the Pavilion into an Orwellian bunker surveilled by sinister-looking Doberman dogs and filled with wire fencing and disturbing performers who would writhe around the floor, screaming and headbanging to music. Two years later, she took over Tate Modern for five nights with *Sex*, where that same strange troupe of performers set things on fire and sang impromptu songs about death. For *Nature Mortes* (2021), staged at the Palais de Tokyo, she invited viewers to confront their mortality as performers moved through empty spaces, filled with light and shadow, or waded through the museum's fountain screaming, singing and sporadically reciting texts. There was a noticeable absence of live performers in 2022's *Avatar II* at London's Sprüth Magers gallery, which centred around themes of nihilism and alienation and featured an ominous deserted locker room, frantic graffiti-like markings and a multi-panel painting of an explosion.

Born in a small village outside of Frankfurt, Imhof was always a rebel. She got kicked out of her English boarding school and spent her twenties immersed in Frankfurt's underground techno scene while studying at the Hochschule für Bildende Künste – Städelschule. At the time she was living in a commune and had formed a punk band, both of which contributed to the sense of subcultural otherness that permeates her work.

Imhof's eldritch aesthetic isn't just limited to her art; it seeps into her personal style too: the often gelled hair that covers her face, the tattoos and all-black wardrobe, full of hardcore band T-shirts and full Balenciaga leather looks. In other words: she is the ultimate modern-day goth.

ARCA

As if from some other dimension, Arca crash-landed onto the scene in 2012 with a series of hypnotic EPs, *Stretch 1* and *Stretch 2*. Before that, Alejandra Ghersi had been performing under a different moniker, Nuuro, in her native Venezuela. Arca's creative output is fluid; with her beautifully grotesque visuals and mind-melting music, her art blurs the boundaries of gender, genre, species and identity. Take her latest endeavour, *KICK* (2020–1), a conceptual multi-album comprising an absurd patchwork of witchy chants, reggaeton beats, pulsating hip hop and dark synths, accompanied by nightmarish visuals that present the artist as part human, part animal and part machine.

Growing up in a conservative gated community in Caracas, she was always at odds with her surroundings and even her own sexuality, which she navigated through her music. She moved to New York aged 17, where she attended NYU and began putting out music as Arca shortly thereafter, carving out a reputation for herself as a true renegade. The last two years have also seen her become something of a fashion muse, having recently starred in campaigns for Calvin Klein, Proenza Schouler and Mugler. With her long, raven hair, signature red lip, and nails sharpened to a point, not to mention typically all-black wardrobe, she's Gen Z's answer to Morticia Addams; a demonic diva for our dystopian world.

COSEY FANNI TUTTI

Cosey Fanni Tutti has made a career out of controversy. Alongside then partner Genesis P-Orridge, Peter 'Sleazy' Christopherson and Chris Carter – fellow members of the COUM Transmissions art collective and experimental music group Throbbing Gristle – she caused outrage when they staged a show at London's Institute of Contemporary Art that comprised a perspex box full of Tutti's used, maggot-infested tampons, a 5ft dildo and a series of magazine spreads featuring her work as a pornographic model. Two years before that, she'd climbed onto a swing at the Oval House Theatre and pissed through a heart-shaped hole in the seat over unsuspecting audience members. Later that evening she and P-Orridge simulated doggy style with giant genitals.

Born Christine Carol Newby, she grew up on a council estate in Hull, where her authoritarian father eventually kicked her out after she refused to get a job. She abhorred the name Christine, and instead went by Cosmosis until 1973, when she changed her name to Cosey Fanni Tutti as a play on the title of Mozart's seminal opera *Così fan tutte*, which can roughly be translated as 'women are like that'. Not that Tutti is like anyone else, at all.

Upon moving to London, Tutti immersed herself in the porn industry; she'd been researching pornographic images for her art and decided to give it a go herself. The one informed the other, with sex, nudity and reclaiming the female form becoming central to her artistic practice. In 1981, she and P-Orridge broke up (she later accused P-Orridge of mental and physical abuse) and Throbbing Gristle disbanded, but not before changing the face of electronic music with their freakish industrial noise, in doing so birthing an entire generation of musical outsiders.

Now in her 70s, Tutti looks the same as she always has: dark berry hair, blunt fringe and mostly pared-back head-to-toe black looks. She still makes art and music, the latter with fellow Throbbing Gristle member and longtime partner Chris Carter. The only difference is that now audiences, including the artistic establishment, are much more receptive. In 2017, the year she staged a COUM retrospective in Hull, she released her spellbinding autobiography *Art Sex Music*, which is currently being turned into a film. Meanwhile, 2022 saw the release of *Re-Sisters*, an exploration of womanhood told through the parallel lives of three unorthodox women: her own, British musician Delia Derbyshire's (best known for her electronic arrangement of the *Doctor Who* theme tune), and that of medieval mystic Margery Kempe. Celebrated for their individualism and refusal to conform to the path laid out for them, they're a lesson to us all, really.

DILARA FINDIKOGLU

Part witch, part rebel, Dilara Findikoglu likes to play with tradition. Drawing on the dichotomies of good and evil, freedom and oppression, virgin and whore, the Turkish-born, London-based designer showed her first collection in a strip club, and her second in a deconsecrated church. Mixing historical dress (corsetry is one of her key signatures) with the tropes of underground youth culture (leather briefs, chaps, slogan T-shirts), her work is an orgy of references that range from Victorian to high goth.

On Planet Dilara, sex and sorcery combine to hypnotic effect, but the work is always political. For the final look of her autumn/winter 23 collection, provocatively named Not a Man's Territory, she sent a model down the runway in a black sheath dress encrusted with Victorian knives. Playing around with the notion of the female body as a battleground to be defended, reclaimed and even weaponized, it was a powerful feminist statement made in reaction to the murder of Iranian student Mahsa Amini in 2023, who was killed after being arrested for not wearing her hijab 'properly'.

Having grown up in a traditional community in Turkey, Findikoglu knows all too well the distinctly male temptation to police women's bodies, as well as the power of fashion to fight back. Part of that fight meant moving to London when she was 19 to study fashion design at Central Saint Martins. In 2015, when she was denied a place to present at the school's prestigious graduate press show, she rallied a group of fellow rebels and staged a guerrilla runway performance outside the official show space. And she's been doing things on her own terms ever since, whether that means speaking out about the struggles of being an independent designer, opting out of Fashion Week altogether, or even in the way she presents herself. Eschewing the understated uniform of most designers today, you'll find her squeezed into a Victorian corset, her petticoat pinned to reveal her thigh, draped in diaphanous lace or dressed head to toe in leather. No matter the situation, she remains unabashedly herself.

DOJA CAT

Doja Cat's story is as much about internet culture as it is about music. Though celebrated for her genre-defying tracks, part of her power lies in her social media presence: her unfiltered streams of consciousness and foul-mouthed diatribes, her Warholian memes and witty retorts to fans. Also thrown into the mix are zoomed-in crops of her face squished under a pair of tights, and candid updates on her recovery from breast reduction surgery.

Born Amala Dlamini, Doja Cat was raised on a diet of memes, sound bites and viral video clips. She had been releasing her own music for more than a decade when, in 2018, she broke the internet with 'Moo!', a song that riffs on bovine puns, which was accompanied by a video that featured the artist eating a beef burger while dressed like a cow. A year later she released 'Say So', sparking a viral TikTok dance challenge. Since then, she has released two groundbreaking albums and won numerous awards including a Grammy and three VMAs.

In 2022, something shifted and she started to embrace a more sepulchral aesthetic, shaving her head and her eyebrows, an event she live-streamed on social media (obvs). A year later, teasing the release of her fourth studio album *Scarlet*, she changed her TikTok profile picture to that of a devilish creature and started posting photos of herself wearing monstrous contact lenses with her limbs stained in blood. She also began covering her body in morbid tattoos; a creature from Fortunio Liceti's *De monstris* (1655) adorns her arm, a scythe festoons her ear and the skeleton of a bat is sprawled across her back. Meanwhile, the videos for singles 'Attention', 'Paint The Town Red' and 'Demons' are replete with gory, horror-inspired visuals.

Doja Cat's approach to style and beauty is just as offbeat. To attend the Schiaparelli spring 2023 couture show, the artist covered her entire face and torso with 30,000 red crystals, while at the 2023 Met Ball she used prosthetics to transform herself into a life-sized version of Karl Lagerfeld's pet cat and meowed her way through her red carpet interviews like the true rebel she is.

EDITH SITWELL

Born in 1887 into one of the great aristocratic English families of the age, Dame Edith Sitwell had a turbulent and traumatic upbringing. There were her mother's bouts of depression and rage, and her father's cruelty and neglect. There was also the pervasive loneliness she experienced growing up in the haunted Renishaw Hall. In spite of this early trauma, or perhaps because of it, Sitwell sought out beauty in the arts, particularly the fraught and lurid writings of French poet Paul Verlaine.

In 1913 she moved to London, where she became immersed in the city's avant-garde scene, and began her own literary career shortly thereafter. Inspired by everything from *commedia dell'arte* and the Ballets Russes to the harrowing atrocities of the Blitz, she created her own language of obscure symbols and references in her poetry and her prose, often paying particular attention to the way words sounded.

But as much as Sitwell was an artist, she was also a muse, sitting for various portraits over the years by the likes of Roger Fry and Cecil Beaton. And like many muses, a certain level of mythology has been created around her: as lore would have it, she would lie in an open coffin before she began her day's work. Much of this mythology can be attributed to her autobiography, *Taken Care Of* (1965), in which she paints a picture of herself as the consummate outsider, born into a life of anguish: the life of a poet. 'I was unpopular with my parents from the moment of my birth. I was in disgrace for being female, and worse, as I grew older, it was obvious that I was not going to conform to my father's standard of beauty,' she writes. Indeed, unlike her mother, who was a great beauty, Sitwell was an unusual sight to behold, thanks to her immense height, crooked nose, large forehead and curved spine. Her parents had tried to correct these with a nose truss and metal braces, the latter of which she used to refer to as her 'bastille'. Instead of trying to hide these perceived abnormalities, she embraced them, particularly in her later years, adding to her statuesque frame and angular features with veils, turbans and striking plumed hats, not to mention layers of fur and brocade and dramatic, oversized jewellery. In short, she was as unorthodox in her style as she was in her writing, and remains a true gothic heroine as a result.

ELVIRA

The dark and stormy creation of Kansas-born Cassandra Peterson, Elvira rose to fame in the 80s thanks to her camp performances and signature spooky style. A former Vegas go-go dancer, she moved to Italy in the 70s, where she began performing with various Italian rock bands until she was introduced to film via the acclaimed Italian director Federico Fellini, who cast her in the semi-autobiographical flick *Roma* (1972). Upon her return to America, she began working as a hostess and glamour model for the Playboy brand, laying the groundwork for her later reincarnation as TV's favourite gothic seductress.

Fast-forward to 1981, and producers from the network KHJ-TV had begun looking for someone to replace Larry Vincent, *aka* Sinister Seymour, as the host for the newly rebooted weekend horror show *Fright Night*. Once talks with Maila Nurmi, the original horror hostess and actress behind 50s pin-up character Vampira, went south, they put out a casting call for another nightmarish vixen, and Peterson promptly answered.

'My late friend, the artist Robert Redding, and I worked together to create Elvira's look,' says Peterson. 'Our parameters from the local TV station were that she must have black hair and a black dress – a prospect that seemed so tired and clichéd to us. We spiced up her look with a little leather, some studs and a jewelled dagger for a 80s metal/punk vibe, and Robert created the makeup based on a photo from a Japanese Kabuki theatre book. The hairstyle was a tribute to one of our favourite singers, Ronnie Spector of the 60s girl group, The Ronettes. We made Elvira's gown as tight and sexy as possible because, you know, ratings.'

Elvira's Movie Macabre aired in September 1981, and Elvira became an overnight success thanks to her captivating combination of rampant sex appeal and self-deprecating humour. Over the years, Elvira evolved from a mere character into a lucrative brand, inspiring a series of spin-off shows, cameo appearances and a cult feature film, *Elvira: Mistress of the Dark* (1988), as well as a slew of action figures, calendars, comic books and Halloween costumes. Now in her 70s, she remains a pop-cultural icon, who is very much part of our collective consciousness today.

ENID COLESLAW

Enid Coleslaw is the sardonic teen protagonist of Daniel Clowes' acclaimed graphic novel *Ghost World*, which was first serialized in his comic book series *Eightball* (1993-7). Eventually published in book form in 1997, *Ghost World* follows the life of the apathetic 18-year-old and her best friend, Rebecca Doppelmeyer, as they float aimlessly around an unnamed dead-end American suburb, hitting up the local diner, record store and thrift shops, and frequenting sex shops for cheap thrills. They hate everything and everyone, from the popular kids to popular culture, and make fun of the various strangers they come into contact with. Having just graduated from high school, they're forced to ponder life's big question of what to do next.

Though she's never described as being a goth, Coleslaw possesses all the trappings of one. She is characterized as droll and maudlin, often playing pranks on people for pure pleasure, in particular a quiet young boy named Josh who she tries to seduce. The foil to Rebecca's 'skinny blonde wasp', she has a boyish crop of inky hair and wears zany thick-rimmed glasses. Her style is as barbed and biting as her *bon mots*, teaming preppy polo shirts in bold prints and lurid hues with combat boots, big leather jackets and a dominatrix cat mask.

In 2001, the misadventures of this teen misanthrope were memorialized in a feature film adaptation directed by Terry Zwigoff and co-written by Clowes. With Scarlett Johansson cast as Rebecca, Coleslaw was brought to life by American actress Thora Birch, who by this point had become something of a poster child for disgruntled teens, having just starred as Kevin Spacey's brilliantly morose and misunderstood daughter Jane Burnham in *American Beauty* (1999). Unlike her comic counterpart, this iteration of Coleslaw is so fraught and contemptuous that even her best friend begins to distance herself from her, pushing Coleslaw into the arms of obscure record collector Seymour, played by Steve Buscemi. In one of cinema's most accurate portrayals of adolescent alienation, there's a poignant scene in which she dyes her hair bright green and calls herself a punk, only to be humiliated in a comic store when told that punk rock is dead, leading her to go home and furiously dye it back to black in a crisis of identity. It's these agonizing moments that make this film so relatable, and why Coleslaw remains one of culture's most important gothic heroines.

ERYKAH BADU

Born in Dallas in 1971, Erykah Badu was raised by a coven of powerful women. There was her mother, grandmothers, godmothers and aunts; healers, carers and guides, all of whom helped to instil a strong sense of self within her. Music was another key feature of her upbringing; the radio was always playing in the background and her grandparents bought her a piano when she was seven, which she taught herself how to play, often staging impromptu performances to anyone who'd listen. She rose to fame in the 90s after being booked to open a show for a then-unknown D'Angelo, and was signed to a record label on the spot.

Badu has never been a goth in the traditional sense. In fact, she rarely wore black, opting instead for vibrant colours and natty prints, which either clash with or complement her signature sky-high headwraps. But there's always been something mystical about her, a shamanic-like aura, something she cultivated through her lyrical references to astrology and spirituality, and in the esoteric and arcane way she presented herself – whether that was by burning incense on stage or by adorning her body with silver rings, bangles and religious ankhs.

Instead of buckling to the more commercial R&B of the moment, Badu helped to birth an entire new genre called Neo Soul, a much richer and authentic counterpoint, which she did with her seminal 1997 album *Baduizm*. Set to a blend of jazz, blues, funk, soul and hip hop, her haunting vocals made her a worldwide success, earning her a slew of Grammys and Soul Train Music Awards.

For the past two decades, Badu has been wafting in and out of public consciousness. But even in those quieter periods, she's never stopped working on her music. A master of reinvention, when lockdown prevented her from touring she'd stage otherworldly concerts from her home, which she'd then broadcast through a special streaming platform named Badutron.

Her look has evolved, too. Now in her 50s, she's begun to embrace a much more eldritch aesthetic, eschewing bold colours in favour of shadowy tones and embracing increasingly macabre makeup: kohl-rimmed eyes, black tears and clumped lashes, livid red eyeshadow and silver grills. Her nails are always sharpened to a point, accentuated further by her stacks of gargantuan rings, while her silhouettes are even more extreme; she's replaced headwraps with towering hats and often experiments with layering and proportion. Badu has spent her entire life ripping up the rule book, and appears to be even more determined to do so with age.

ETHEL CAIN

Ethel Cain is the bewitching alter ego of 24-year-old singer-songwriter Hayden Anhedönia. As if straight out of some piece of Southern Gothic fiction, the character came to Anhedönia as a vision back in 2018: a diaphanous figure dressed in ivory with long, dark hair.

Cain was first introduced to the world in 2021 via Anhedönia's breakout EP *Inbred* – a witchy blend of pop that dealt with themes of sex and violence. Until this point, Anhedönia had been putting her ethereal music out online under the moniker White Silas to an ever-growing fanbase. It wasn't until her debut album, *Preacher's Daughter* (2022), that we got the full story. Initially conceived as a screenplay, Cain's twisted tale begins in 1991: having escaped her strict religious upbringing in the Deep South, she soon fell into the clutches of a tumultuous relationship, one that descended into kidnapping, addiction, prostitution, death and, of course, cannibalization – as it sometimes does.

Like Cain, Anhedönia grew up in a strict Southern Baptist household in rural Florida, where she was home-schooled by her deacon father. As a trans woman, Anhedönia's relationship with religion is complex, and she left the church when she was 16. It is through music that she finds catharsis. Haunting and melancholic, Anhedönia's unique body of work is inspired by the mix of country music, Gregorian chants and gospel she grew up listening to, while her gothic visuals are an homage to her favourite horror movies.

Although steeped in nostalgia, Anhedönia's aesthetic is also distinctly modern. She recently cut her hair to just below the shoulders and often alternates romantic prairie dresses with vintage T-shirts and ripped jeans. For her debut performance at Coachella, she wore a red-and-white cheerleader's outfit by Givenchy. In fact, fashion plays a key role in the singer's creative practice; as well as fronting Givenchy's autumn/winter 2022 campaign, she made her runway debut for Miu Miu and Eckhaus Latta at the spring/summer 2023 shows.

For the past four years, Anhedönia has been submerged in the character of Ethel Cain. Precisely where one ends and the other begins is unclear. An obvious difference is that where Cain met a tragic end (yes, it's confusing, but let's just go with it), Anhedönia is very much still alive. Moving forward, she now plans to focus on the story of Cain's mother. Until then, Cain remains a vital part of Anhedönia's identity, a vessel through which she can navigate her creativity, come to terms with her fraught past and ultimately lay the foundations for her future.

FKA TWIGS

Watching one of FKA twigs' hypnotic performances is like succumbing to the powers of a snake charmer; she captivates her audiences with her impossible contortions and enigmatic ballads.

Born Tahliah Debrett Barnett, she acquired her nickname 'twigs' after the way her limbs would crack during dance practice, and added the FKA later to distinguish herself from the musical duo The Twigs. A self-proclaimed misfit, twigs, who is of Jamaican, Spanish and English descent, grew up in a small village in Gloucestershire, where she discovered an early affinity with opera, theatre and dance. After moving to London to work as a backup dancer, in 2012 she released her groundbreaking *EP1*, which featured a host of experimental tracks. A year later, she put out the equally arresting follow-up *EP2*.

An intoxicating blend of raw vocals, avant-garde pop and futuristic R&B, her sonic landscape defies genre, and is often accompanied by a tableau of unsettling visuals, like the bruised head the artist Jesse Kanda created for the cover of her debut album *LP1* (2014), while her performances mix elements of pole dancing, sword fighting and martial arts. A lot of her work is conceptual; for her second studio album, *Magdalene* (2019), she inhabited the much-maligned character of Mary Magdalene, through which she was able to express ideas about love, loss, pain and spirituality.

FKA twigs' approach to beauty and style is just as alluring; she constantly wears vintage pieces with hooded elements in an array of earthy tones, which she combines with layers of gold jewellery and extraterrestrial facial markings. A constant shapeshifter, it is her outright refusal to conform, combined with her utterly mesmerizing brand of theatrics, which ultimately makes her synonymous with the goth experience.

GABBRIETTE BECHTEL

Model of the moment Gabbriette Bechtel looks more likely to down a vial of blood than she does a green juice – yet it's via the latter that she gets her morning fix. The ultimate paradox, from the outset she embodies the quintessential 90s goth. With her liquorice locks, smudged charcoal eyes and trademark lobotomized stare, she oozes a stygian glamour. Then there's the leather trousers, corsets and biker jackets, the crucifixes, chokers and tattoos. But there's this whole other side to her, too; nestled in between the sullen thirst traps, her Instagram is peppered with recipes for romanesco salad, golden beetroots and grain-free bread. In one viral video, she recreates upscale LA health food spot Erewhon's famous vegan blackout cake, which she filmed in her own kitchen. It's precisely this tension between granola goddess and gothic priestess that makes her so alluring – a testament to the fact that you can be both dark and healthy at the same time.

Born in Orange County, Bechtel never really felt like she fit in. Half Mexican, half German, she stood out among the sea of perky blondes at her school and would often be found skulking around the dance theatre, daydreaming about her future as a professional dancer. In 2013, a spot as a backup dancer in the music video for Dev Hynes's 'Chamakay' brought her to LA, where she formed a band called Nasty Cherry (now defunct) and signed to a model agency a few years later.

Fast-forward to today and the 26-year-old represents a new type of beauty that eschews traditional notions of perfection in favour of something much more unique. In the last year alone, she's gone from an unknown face to being *the* face of brands such as Bottega Veneta, Skims and Heaven by Marc Jacobs. And as goth continues to be embraced by the mainstream, she's showing no signs of slowing down.

HELENA BONHAM CARTER

The descendant of a former UK prime minister, Helena Bonham Carter was born into a prominent political family but instead found her footing in the arts. While she may have risen to fame playing pretty period ingénues like Lucy Honeychurch in *A Room with a View* (1985), it's her turns as dark and twisted types for which she is best known. So far, in her illustrious career, she's played a smattering of wicked witches, an evil Queen of Hearts, two tragic brides (one from beyond the grave, another fast approaching it), a sinister baker with a taste for cannibalic pies, and a psychiatrist who deals in all things undead – most of which have been part of her ongoing collaboration with director Tim Burton, the great gothic auteur and Bonham Carter's ex-husband, with whom she worked on *Big Fish* (2003), *Corpse Bride* (2005), *Sweeney Todd: The Demon Barber of Fleet Street* (2007), *Alice in Wonderland* (2010) and *Dark Shadows* (2012).

Bonham Carter celebrates the eccentric misfit and comes alive in roles that pertain to death, imbuing them with a kind of dark romance that makes them unexpectedly appealing. Take the beautiful but unhinged Bellatrix Lestrange in the *Harry Potter* (2001–10) series or the exquisitely maudlin Miss Havisham in *Great Expectations* (2012).

There's a powerful synergy between Bonham Carter and the roles she inhabits, so much so that it's often hard to tell where her characters end and where she begins – well, apart from the murder and black magic. Breaking free of the stereotypical 'woman of a certain age' trope, Bonham Carter rocks the boat sartorially with her ghostly white complexion and bird's nest hair, faintly stained teeth and signature witch-like cackle. Not to mention her brilliantly unconventional look, which is so often the subject of public derision; a mishmash of Victorian mourning dress, Vivienne Westwood corsetry, big boots and taffeta skirts. Ultimately, what is so alluring about Bonham Carter is that she does things on her own terms, whether that's the roles she plays or the way she puts herself together, both of which have been emboldened by age. She's a lesson to us all.

ISABELLA BLOW

To commemorate the life and death of fashion's rarest, most exotic bird, Isabella Blow, the designer Alexander McQueen and milliner Philip Treacy staged a funeral that people would talk about for years to come. Her body was driven to Gloucester Cathedral in the most gothic of hearses, a traditional Victorian horse-drawn funeral carriage strewn with white gardenias and adorned with a hat in the shape of a ship. She was as glamorous in death as she had been in life.

Blow always had a flair for drama, something that manifested through her surreal and often outrageous style choices. She used clothes as if they were armour, and often used armour – her favourite was medieval chainmail – as if it were clothes. Even her statement red lips and severe 20s-style bob became part of her artistic expression.

Born in Cheshire, Blow's story reads like some foreboding gothic fairy tale. Growing up in the shadow of Doddington Hall, the Delves-Broughton family's former ancestral home, her childhood was struck by tragedy after witnessing her younger brother drown in a lake. Unable to cope with the grief, her mother walked out on the family and Blow was sent away to boarding school. It was during her 20s that she moved to America and began working at American *Vogue* under Anna Wintour, until a job in *Tatler*'s fabled halls drew her back to England. Steeped in theatre and fantasy, the fashion stories she created there were as witty as they were subversive, often turning tradition on its head in a way that would titillate, if not shock, the magazine's upper-crust readership.

In 1989 she married the gallerist Detmar Blow in a spectacularly gothic wedding, to which she wore a purple velvet robe, gold headdress and medieval wimple. Soon after, the couple moved into Hilles, a sprawling Arts and Crafts house jam-packed with William Morris tapestries, suits of armour and other medieval ephemera.

Throughout the 90s, Blow started turning her attention to nurturing talent, taking designers like Philip Treacy,

Hussein Chalayan and Alexander McQueen under her wing. She famously bought the last's entire graduate collection and invited him to work out of her London apartment. It came as a complete shock, then, when Blow was excluded from McQueen's new role at Givenchy, a deal that Blow purportedly helped to broker, which sent her into a decline. She started dressing in black, wearing elements of traditional Victorian mourning dress and spoke a lot about death, particularly her own. After several suicide attempts, Blow died in 2007. But her contributions to both British fashion and the gothic canon remain everlasting.

Chapter VI:
The goths and goth-coded:
in their words, part I

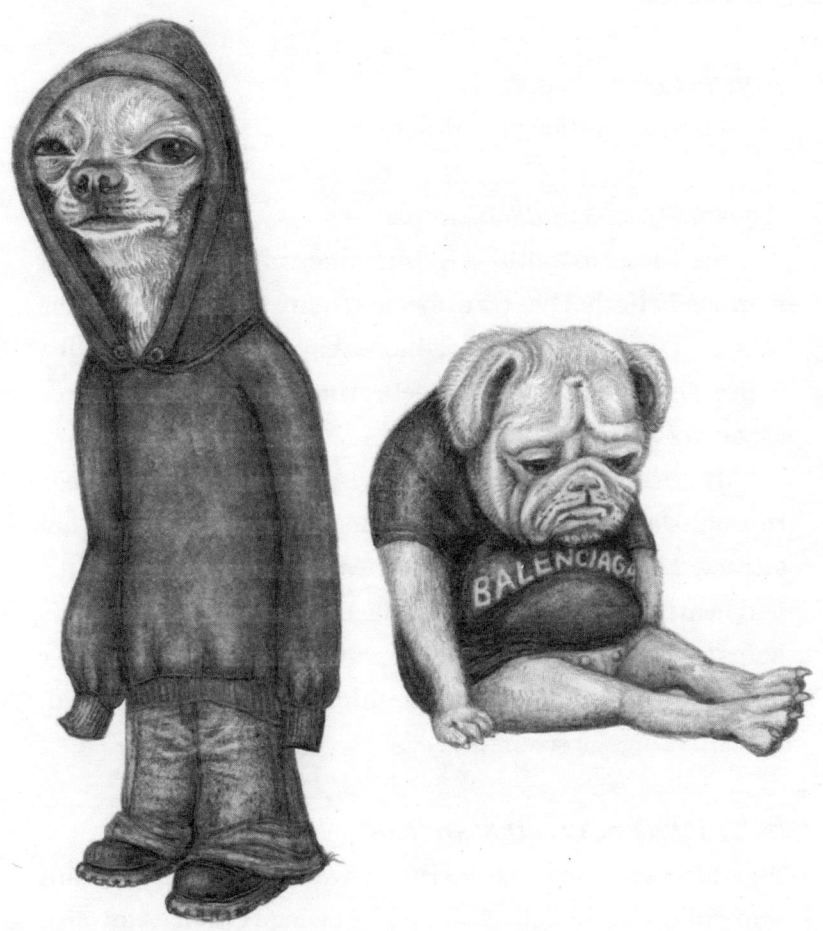

Amelia Gray, model
'Gothic style makes me feel like the most powerful version of myself. It's almost a protective armour to me. Without it, I don't feel like me.'

Anjelica Huston, actress
'Goth is a celebration of darkness.'

Aryuna Tardis, makeup artist
'For me, the term "goth" is the definition of self-expression, it is an aesthetic that has transformed from a subculture into the masses. The goth lifestyle is all about embracing individuality, expressing creativity and celebrating the beauty in darker aspects of life.

'My creativity is the art of pain. By expressing my feelings through dark aesthetics, I learn more about myself. I am not attracted to talking about happiness. I talk about suffering, and heartbreak, and reflect on the theme of pain in art. This helps people not to close their eyes to the dark sides of their minds, thereby exposing their vulnerabilities to the world. Isn't this a sign of strength?'

Betsy Johnson, creative director
'I've always worn black since I was a teenager. It's not something I've thought about. It's just what I gravitate toward. Maybe there's a psychoanalytical reason for that. I've never referred to myself as a goth.'

Brenda Weischer, aka Brenda Hashtag, fashion editor
'Growing up, I was never part of any subculture. I tried to be an emo, but my parents weren't really supportive of my emo lifestyle. I have always looked at goths as kind of a mysterious phenomenon. I was always fascinated by the fashion, but not so much by the music. I was never really into wearing colour, which is partly just because I'm very pale with a pink undertone. I just don't think it looks good on me. When I was about 15, I cut out most colours from my life until eventually I was left with just a black and white wardrobe. I've always been fascinated by finding a uniform where everything matches and everything goes together and you don't really have to think, because I feel like we have so many choices nowadays and we waste so much time trying to figure out what to wear.

'There are a lot of people that are super loud and really smiley, and we often find out they're actually sad when they're alone. It's the exact same with fashion: you see people in the most joyful clothes, and sometimes they're actually not so joyful. What I find with people all dressed in black is maybe it's a very hard shell, and you seem kind of unapproachable, and for sure I use the black clothes as kind of an armour, you know, not to be approached or to be left alone, which sounds maybe really sad, but to me, it's just kind of a safety net. What I have often found is that the people who dress in black, whatever you might have thought of them on first impression was actually not true. In reality, they're super kind and super loving and very cheerful.

'I have been called a goth many times in my life, but I

don't think I really fit into that category. I just happen to wear only black. But it's the colour that makes me feel most confident. Within fashion, you try to find the silhouette that fits you, the colour that suits you the best, whatever makes you feel your best so that you act your best in a certain way. So fashion is a really important part of my life in order to represent myself.'

Cassandra Peterson, actress

'To me, goth is a subculture of people who grew up feeling like they didn't fit in or were somehow "different" or overlooked. The goths created a look and lifestyle that made them stand out, gave them a "home", and supplied an outlet for their creativity. I believe their deepest, darkest inner feelings are reflected on the outside, through their hair, makeup and dress.'

Christina Ricci, actress

'I have never really been able to put myself in a category or label myself. I don't love colour, I love more luxe fabrics and I also am a person who genuinely does not like the sun. It gives me horrible headaches. My mum says I've been like this since I was a child. So I think naturally, I found more beauty in things that happen at night and the moon. And because I don't like the sun, I'm always usually really pale, and certain things just work better with a person who is always really pale and I have dark hair. I guess if I'm being really honest, I don't like looking like what's popular or looking like other people.

'It's a reaction to the pressure. You think, "I'm never going to look like that person that I'm supposed to try to look like.

So guess what? I'm going to look like the exact opposite." It's a rebellion to what we've been told we should be.

'I wouldn't call myself a goth. I have an interest in things that are supposedly goth. But for me, what defines goth is seeing the beauty in things that traditionally have not been seen as beautiful.'

Cosey Fanni Tutti, artist

'I've never been part of the mainstream. I've felt no affinity with it as my interests, music and art have been regarded as odd, mysterious or transgressive. I function best in the shadows, so I favour wearing black or dark colours, they feel right, and don't draw too much attention. I'm free of unwanted distractions, unless the occasion, private or public, warrants otherwise. It's about freedom of choice.

'I don't really think of goth as having one meaning. I have friends who would be called goth but to me, they are people I share interests with. Because our music has focused on the esoteric, fetishistic and dark issues, it has fallen into the goth category as well as others. As Carter Tutti, Chris and I performed at the Wave-Gotik-Treffen festival in Germany and saw the most incredible and diverse display of goth style. Clothes, makeup, and whatever constitutes our outer appearance make an important statement, either bold or subtle. It's about communication.'

Chapter VII:
Goths all grown up: notes on style

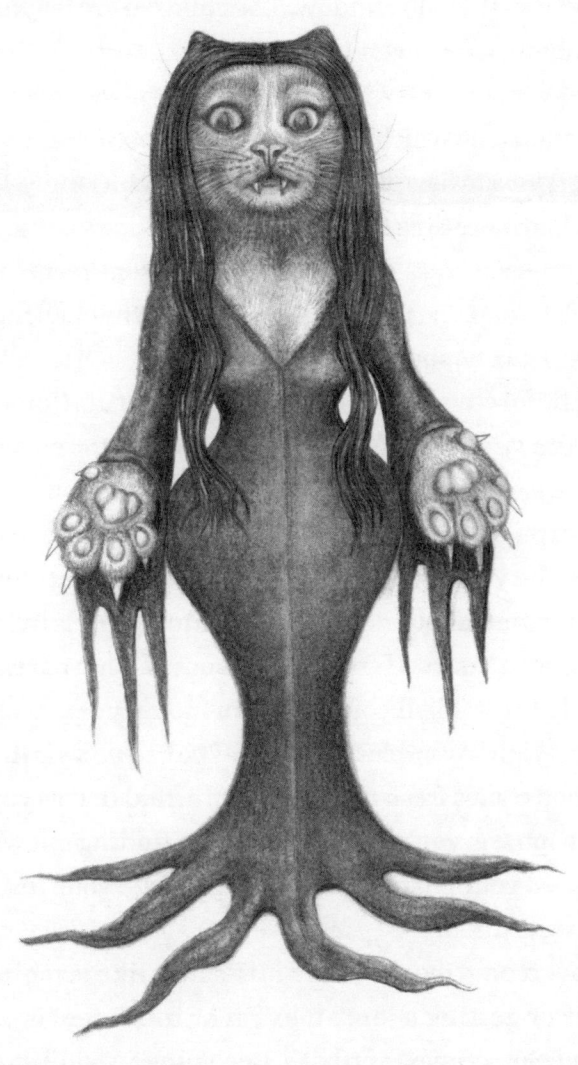

There's a scene in *Addams Family Values* (1993) in which Morticia Addams and her husband, Gomez, are sharing a romantic moonlit moment in the family graveyard. As they lean in to kiss each other they are interrupted by the shrieking sound of a shattering window. The children are playing with cannonballs in a never-ending game of torture. Gomez is concerned about his wife and the many plates which she's been spinning, to which she laments, 'I'm just like any modern woman trying to have it all. Loving husband, a family. It's just, I wish I had more time to seek out the dark forces and join their hellish crusade.' As a mother of two, it's a sentiment to which I can relate, and one that sums up many of the challenges our goth must face as she enters adulthood.

But before we get onto those, congratulations are in order. You've made it. You've emerged from the chrysalis of adolescence (albeit not completely unscathed). Blighted by growing pains and changing body parts, you've managed to resist the youthful urge to blend in, learning to embrace your intramural outsider instead. More crucially, you've emancipated yourself from the bosom of your parents and are ready to establish yourself as an independent woman in your own right. Wimples off to you! The bad news is that with adulthood comes fresh new hells. I'm afraid that as you enter this new phase, you're still no closer to finding out who you are or what your purpose is in life. Although your Instagram might beg to differ.

To overcome most of life's obstacles, like learning how to drive or getting a job, an exam or interview is usually required. Sometimes even both. Becoming an adult, however, is something that just happens to you. There's no practice round or chance to revise or prep. There's no job specification either, to provide a framework for what exactly it is you're going up against. Instead, you're being thrown in the deep end of the swamp and you've barely learned how to swim – yet somehow you're expected to know how to pay your taxes, ask for a raise, hand in your resignation, build a career, get a mortgage, get a house, freeze your eggs, weather fertility scares or IVF, navigate parent Whatsapp groups, handle in-laws, help with homework, not swear in front of your kids, keep on top of medical check-ups, not say the wrong thing, deal with loss, grief and worsening hangovers, deal with diagnoses of depression, anxiety and adult ADHD, get your head around the encroaching menopause and that funny flabby bit that appears and won't leave, accept yourself, love yourself, but also do better, be better, work harder, earn more, get more followers, embrace your lines, wrinkles and greys, but also experiment with Botox, lasers and microneedling, stay positive, be mindful and always remember to practise gratitude. You also need to be a good employee, boss, parent or partner and put something out into the world that you're actually proud of, all the while dealing with raging imposter syndrome and the fact that you're not like other women, all shiny, perky and happy. You're difficult and dark and drawn to the macabre. You may be older, but those feelings never go away.

The best advice? Fake it till you make it. It sounds trite, but eventually, things will start to fall into place and you'll realize you've been doing it all on your own this whole time, just under the guise of making it up. A lot of this comes down to looking the part. Of course, honing your wardrobe isn't going to pay the bills or cure your anxiety or depression, but it will afford you a firmer grip on who you are. Where style was once a weapon to be wielded in the face of parents, teachers and the patriarchy, it now becomes the building blocks of your identity, a way to navigate the pangs of imposter syndrome and feelings of self-loathing and inadequacy. Because it's only when you have some semblance of self that you can begin to tackle all those other problems.

After the birth of my son, I went through a bit of an existential crisis. A small bomb went off inside my head and I realized I had no idea what I was doing. I was 28, which isn't young, but I still thought of myself as a teenager. That's not to say that motherhood and adulthood are mutually exclusive – they just happened to converge at the same time for me. So, to get me through this next phase, I realized I needed to start dressing the part. I needed a new sartorial language that allowed me to stay true to my gothic sensibilities, but would also help me convey a sense that I was now all grown up; a style with which I could meet other parents at the school gate, communicate authoritatively with teachers, return to work with a set of new non-negotiable boundaries, as opposed to taking on more than I could handle (my usual default), and meet with lawyers to draw up scary grown-up things like my will.

Whereas borrowing from the gothic canon was previously about looking hot, cool, scary and ugly, all at the same time – an urgent expression of your otherness and of the searing angst within – now it's about consolidating your identity as you climb the undulating hills of adulthood on your own terms. This requires nuance, restraint and a certain level of subtlety. It also calls for buying lots of incredibly similar-looking items (the essentials) to create signature looks. That's not to say you've suddenly become all conservative. It's just that there are ways of communicating your outsider status without donning a dog collar and Doc Martens. Think less Siouxsie Sioux and more Susie Cave – it's a quieter gothic glamour that you're after here, or a pared-back stygian futurism in the manner of creative director Martina Tiefenthaler and her sardonic play on silhouettes. It's not about the hardcore shock tactics of the Batcave era, all PVC harnesses and fishnet bodies. Although there's certainly still a place for these in your arsenal. You can (and should!) still be experimental, it's just about being overall more refined. Indeed, instead of sex-shop latex, look to the sleazy cool of emerging designers like Betsy Johnson or Mowalola, whose oversized leather trenches and navel-grazing biker jackets, respectively, add that extra bit of elevation. Instead of Army surplus boots, sink your teeth into some embellished platform kicks from Japanese designer Junya Watanabe.

There's another thing happening here. By this point, our goth has woken up to the world of high fashion, along with her newfound personal spending power. No longer confined to pillaging charity shops or late-night negotiations on Depop, her pockets now run a little deeper, and the bright lights of Dover Street Market have been calling her name. Instead of searching for style tribes, these days she's hunting for individual brands and designers with whom she can align herself. Not just contemporary fashion, either. This goth worships at the temple of Alexander McQueen; she's done her research and knows her Highland Rape from her The Widows of Culloden. She has also studied how the industry's greatest muses – Amanda Harlech, Isabella Blow and Daphne Guinness – put themselves together in the late 90s and early noughties, using a dark sartorial language to carve out powerful identities for themselves. Harlech with her sharp tailoring, black Chanel tweed and full taffeta skirts; Blow with her monochromatic houndstooth skirt suits and surreal hats; Guinness with her breastplates and gargantuan heel-less boots.

But that isn't to say your wardrobe needs to exclusively be high-end. On the contrary; the idea is to invest in a few timeless and expertly curated pieces that set you apart from the pack and which you can use as a way of subverting the unspoken dress codes of the adult world, whether that's by wearing Balenciaga's directional athleisure wear on the school run, Yohji Yamamoto tailoring to work or a vintage John Galliano midnight slip to a summer wedding. In fact, wearing black when it isn't appropriate is one of the most satisfying acts of rebellion out there.

Buying vintage or second-hand is an excellent way to tap into high fashion. Not only does it give you access to the ghosts of fashion past, but it's also so much more affordable than buying things fresh off the runway and goes some way to offsetting your carbon footprint. After all, our planet is not well. If the prices are still too prohibitive, there are great rental platforms out there and you can always resell purchases once you're done with them.

Don't be afraid to mix things up, either; one day you might be deconstructed in 90s-era Ann Demeulemeester, the next, you're dialling up the drama in Dilara Findikoglu corsetry or giving vampire girl-boss like fanged beauty Miriam Blaylock in camp horror flick *The Hunger* (1983), with 80s-inspired power suits and strategically placed leather. Experiment with masculine and feminine codes, too, with exaggerated proportions and asymmetric silhouettes. And play with different style periods: wear riding gear with Lycra, and granny twin sets with 30s lace. Styles meld seamlessly when all the components are black. But don't be afraid to bring in colour: reds, purples and animal prints, dark vampy tones that speak to your inner vixen. You can also get away with pastel hues during the summer months by mixing 40s silk nightgowns with Edwardian blouses, antique lace and Simone Rocha's hauntingly beautiful spun-sugar separates. Or by channelling original 70s sorceress Stevie Nicks for a more hippy-goth look with bell-sleeved dresses, skinny scarfs and winged crop tops. Welcome to your White Witch era. Think the *Virgin Suicides'* ghostly Lisbon sisters or the girls of *Picnic at Hanging Rock* (1975) – only now all grown up.

Coming of age as a goth is a painful experience; navigating adulthood as one is that much harder. The stakes are higher, the responsibilities manifold and you can't blame your mistakes on youthful naivety. The good news is that you have the independent-mindedness of goth to help carve out your own character and identity from which confidence and self-respect spring. In other words, it gives you the balls to do things your way and to look good while doing it.

STYLE CHECKLIST: THE ESSENTIALS

The tabi boot

When Belgian designer Martin Margiela first launched the tabi boot back in 1988, he had models walk through red paint so as to leave strange, bloodied hoof marks on the catwalk in their wake. Not quite man, but not quite beast either; if the devil himself made footprints, they would look a lot like this. Margiela didn't come up with the design. Its cleft shape can be traced back to 15th-century Japan, where split-toe socks were worn to encourage mental and physical balance. Initially the preserve of the upper crust, by the 20th century rubber soles had been added for outdoor activities, and the tabi, or *jika-tabi* as they were now known, had become the dominant workwear shoe.

Margiela had become fascinated with the design after a trip to Japan, and decided to base a boot on them for his debut show. At the time, the design was seen as so radical that only one cobbler would take on the task of making them: Mr Zagato. Fast-forward to today and the tabi comes in myriad forms, from ballet pumps to brogues, but it is the boot which remains the most iconic, in its morbid suspension of reality. Both horrifying and yet strangely hypnotic, it's feminine and formal but with a transgressive Mr Tumnus twist, making it the ultimate shoe for the working goth to hoof around in, on her daily cemetery/Starbucks trip.

Balenciaga athleisure wear

In 2021, Balenciaga's creative director Demna escorted Kim Kardashian to the Met Ball in custom Balenciaga looks. Dressed head-to-toe in black and with their faces concealed by masks, they appeared as silhouettes of themselves. Here was the most famous woman in the world, hidden in plain sight on one of the biggest, most glamorous occasions of the fashion calendar. It was irreverent, iconoclastic and totally genius. It was also incredibly goth. Even more brilliant was the fact that this red-carpet look was essentially cobbled out of a T-shirt and matching jersey bodysuit.

By this point, Demna had been at Balenciaga for six years and had already established jersey as part of his style signatures. Recontextualizing this humble fabric as a luxury material, he elevated basic athleisure wear – sweatpants, joggers, leggings, T-shirts, sweatshirts and hoodies – through unusual proportions, architectural design and high concept ideas, like a T-shirt sewn onto a shirt or high-waisted leggings with built-in boots.

It's easy to think of gothic style as stuffy, rigid and arcane – the mothball mustiness that comes with buying vintage and the richness of materials like velvet, lace and leather, all layered together, but it doesn't have to be that way. In fact, there's a whole style lexicon out there that reconsiders goth as a profoundly modern, if not futuristic phenomenon, which is exactly what Demna does with his black-clad ergonomic designs. It's a form of normcore for those who don't want to blend in. A way for you to work out and wear black, be sporty and sad at the same time. It's health goth, but high fashion.

By adding one of Demna's patched track pants or oversized T-shirts to your arsenal, you can instantly update your look. And they're versatile, too – throw on a cropped hoodie for the school run before heading out to the gym, then dress it up later with a pair of heels and sharp tailoring. Consider creative director Betsy Johnson and the way she pairs the brand's oversized T-shirts with second-skin leggings and razor-sharp boots. Fresh and directional, it takes the codes of the street, refines them and places them within a luxury context. You can play with masculine and feminine codes, too. Take German artist Anne Imhof, who lends a cool androgyny to Demna's lugubrious designs by mixing tracksuit bottoms with his sculptural tailoring. Something to bear in mind for when you're feeling more Gomez than Morticia.

Yohji Yamamoto tailoring

Ever since 19th-century French actress Sarah Bernhardt sent shock waves through Paris in a custom-made trouser suit, women's tailoring has been imbued with a sense of anarchy. Throughout the 30s, 40s and 50s, masculine silhouettes confounded expectations of gender; in 1966, Yves Saint Laurent revolutionized eveningwear with his Le Smoking tuxedo suit. In the 80s, large shoulder pads communicated independence and invited respect. Today, tailoring is largely seen as a staple, but there are ways to tap into its discordant power.

Yohji Yamamoto enters the chat. A master tailor, Yamamoto has been shattering convention with his avant-garde designs and almost exclusive palette of black since he showed his first collection in Tokyo back in 1977. Deconstructing classic tailoring with his intricate draping, raw edges, precise cut-outs and loose shapes, he takes the politeness of formal dressing and undoes it completely. The result is fluid, elegant, poetic and punk. Whether it's a gabardine collarless overcoat or baggy suit trousers with side pleats worn with an asymmetric double-fronted jacket, incorporating an element of Yamamoto's tailoring into your arsenal equates to a subtle act of sedition.

The John Galliano slip dress

John Galliano is a master storyteller. Whether referencing 20s femmes fatales or French Revolution libertines, the British designer's propensity for fantasy and theatre knows no bounds. He doesn't just stage shows, he invents parallel universes. Throughout his tenure at Christian Dior and at the helm of his own namesake brand, he often drew on gothic characters and themes: sex, death, violence, religion, Siouxsie Sioux, Joan of Arc, Lucrezia Borgia, the Marquis de Sade. He would weave dresses out of cobwebs and silk slips out of shadows. For his spring/summer 2006 couture collection at Christian Dior, models were sent down the runway wearing giant crucifixes and had blood dripping from their just-bitten necks. The following season, models were swathed in medieval armour and full-skirted latex dresses laden with occult symbols, and had bat-like wings coming out of their hair.

There's no better way to unleash your inner freak than by going all-out in Galliano at the school gate, but for those shrinking belladonnas among you, a subtle way to channel the macabre is by investing in one of the designer's simple black bias-cut slips, which you can source online. A whisper of a thing, it can be fashioned out of lace, silk, chiffon or decadent velvet devoré. Keep it casual by throwing on a cardigan or a cropped crew-neck jumper. Alternatively, lean into the drama with an opera coat and a multi-strand choker for the ultimate modern-day mistress of the underworld look. If in doubt, Google images of Amanda Harlech in the 90s.

If you can't get your hands on the real deal, look to 30s bias-cut dresses, which are what Galliano based many of his designs on. In fact, there's something talismanic about wearing a dress that's nearly a hundred years old; it lends an antiquity and spiritual magnetism to your look, which is part of what goth is all about.

An Alaïa bodycon

What would Morticia Addams be without her slinky black dress? It's a vital item for any goth as she manoeuvres her way through adulthood. The key here is to avoid pastiche. You don't want it to look like you've fished it out of a dressing-up box or ordered it on Amazon Prime. This isn't Halloween. What you want is a tight-fitting number that expertly accentuates the curves of your body. It's about oozing dark glamour and sultry femininity without being gimmicky or overly conformist. Which is where Azzedine Alaïa comes in.

Dubbed the King of Cling, the Tunisian designer and master pattern-cutter rose to fame in the 80s thanks to his meticulously constructed body-conscious creations. He was constantly experimenting with new fabrics and worked by draping material directly onto live models. One technique involved using bands of stretch jersey to expertly mould the body without restricting it.

For Alaïa, the job of a dress was to become a kind of second skin, a daring celebration of the female form, which is exactly the kind of thing you need in your wardrobe, whether that's a vintage crochet dress with dramatic bell sleeves by the designer himself, which you can find on Vestiaire, or a spooky floor-skimming, hooded chenille number by Pieter Mulier, who was appointed creative director of the brand after the designer died in 2017.

Ann Demeulemeester everyday wear

Patti Smith was never a goth in the traditional sense, but she wasn't totally dissimilar to them either, and that's in no small part due to Belgian designer Ann Demeulemeester, whose dark and brooding designs she's been wearing for the last few decades. A key member of the Antwerp Six, a group of Belgian designers who graduated in 1986 from Antwerp's Royal Academy of Fine Art, Demeulemeester rose to prominence in the 90s for her funereal take on androgynous dressing. Early designs were non-conformist and nonchalant; loose tailoring and shirts worn off the shoulder, drop-stitch sweaters and chunky shoes, but they became more romantic and individualist over the years, with barbed-wire detailing, coq feathers, hooded dresses and combat boots.

Never one to buckle to trends (Demeulemeester herself has dressed exclusively in black since she was a teenager), her stygian brand of glamour is uniquely her own, and despite retiring in 2013 she remains involved with the brand today, now helmed by creative director Stefano Gallici. Away from the theatre of the runway show, what has remained a constant since the brand's inception are Demeulemeester's everyday staples: tank tops, column dresses and slouchy shirts. There's also the deconstructed tailoring, lightweight sweaters and languid silk skirts. Whether vintage or contemporary, overtly feminine or more androgynous, these items are an essential part of any goth's armoury. Alternatively, take a leaf out of Patti Smith's punk playbook and invest in a pair of Demeulemeester's beautifully crafted leather combat boots. Knee-high or ankle. With laces or without.

Tom Ford bondage gear

You may have grown up a bit, but you haven't lost your sense of fun or danger. Where before you were buying bondage from a local sex shop, consider buying it courtesy of Tom Ford-era Gucci. For his spring/summer 1998 collection, the Texan designer sent black-clad models down his runway in a series of form-fitting pencil skirts and matching stretch fabric long-sleeve and vest tops. On the surface, it was business as usual, but upon closer inspection, you could see patent leather straps with shiny logo buckles peeking out of waistlines and at the shoulders mimicking the effect of exposed lingerie. It was giving sexy secretary with a sordid twist. Officecore, but make it dirty. The previous season, he rounded out his show with a sling of long black dresses replete with patent leather harnesses around the neck and wrap-around miniskirts with patent leather belts. In fact, harness detailing and strategically placed straps, strings and buckles, along with other illicit tropes like leather, cut-outs, bandages and spiked dominatrix heels, featured throughout Ford's tenure as he looked to bondage to inform his hyper-sexual language.

Powerful and subversive, sourcing some vintage Tom Ford pieces online is an easy way to sex up your look without straying from the gothic tradition – you just have to overlook the price tag. But remember there are deals to be made and bargains to be had. And if not, there are ways of recreating the look for less, you just need to get creative.

Alexander McQueen anything

Of all the gothic artists out there, British designer Alexander McQueen was the most rigorous. His 1992 graduate collection was named after Jack the Ripper and he used to sew locks of human hair (his own) into the lining of his clothes. Steeping his collections in the codes of gothic horror, throughout his career he transformed models into monsters, and muses such as Isabella Blow and Daphne Guinness into eldritch works of art.

For his 1997 couture collection for Givenchy, *memento mori* jewellery was made out of vulture claws, while resin vulture skulls (skulls were one of his key motifs) perched on models' shoulders. Elsewhere, chokers were fashioned out of

Victorian-style jet beading and what looked like ravens' wings, while other models wore funereal black lace veils. Even more disturbing, for his autumn/winter 1998 collection at his own brand, McQueen recalled the burning figure of Joan of Arc by sending models in medieval chainmail and shimmering red sequin gowns down a fiery runway with crimson contact lenses and ghostly white makeup. And finally, for his spring/ summer 2001 collection, he conjured an image of an asylum, with models wrapped in head bandages fingering the walls of a mirrored glass box, while at the centre was a grotesque masked figure hooked up to breathing tubes and lying naked on a horned bed.

McQueen continued to harness his singular vision of gothic beauty until he died in 2010. If you can tap into that by acquiring something from the master himself, whether that's a sharply tailored pencil skirt or leather guardsman jacket, you're in pretty good stead.

NOTES ON BEAUTY

Growing up, my beauty choices were dictated by a deadly mix of anarchy and anxiety, insecurity and youthful irreverence. As a result, they were bold, blatant and in your face. As I got older, however, I realized that I didn't need to be so staunch in my refusal to fit in. Instead, I could access a level of chicness and refinement without looking boring, conformist or beige. I could do adult things, like get a blow dry, go for a facial or wear red lipstick, without sacrificing what it was that made me different. More specifically, I could channel a grown-up sense of femininity and still retain an element of darkness and strength.

Inspired by sombre sirens Morticia Addams, Lily Munster, Elvira and Vampira, I started experimenting with a bold red lip. Opting for crimson tones in matte textures, I would accentuate the Cupid's bow with lip liner to look like gothic cathedral arches for a dramatic twist. I began to refine my eyes, too, with feline flicks and artfully rendered (as opposed to haphazardly smeared) smokey hues. I also broadened my colour palette to include poppy, copper and burgundy on both the upper and lower lids, so much so that a rouge eye has become something of a signature look, rendered in shimmery, matte and sometimes glossy textures. It's giving conjunctivitis chic.

The point I'm making here isn't to rush out and buy a load of red beauty products, but rather to figure out what works for you and then finesse it. If in those coming-of-age years, beauty is a vehicle for creativity and expression, transformation and exploration, in this next period, it is a way of distinguishing and consolidating your individual identity. Taking the rebelliousness of youth and refining it to create something lasting and unique. The reason those macabre matriarchs Morticia Addams and Lily Munster are so ingrained in collective consciousness is because their look was so specific. This isn't about copying them verbatim – far from it – but rather using them as examples of women who derive a certain sense of confidence and power through the vocabulary of goth.

Apart from an unwise attempt at balayage, I've kept my hair the same black coffee hue it's always been. Only it's a lot sleeker and cared for than it was in the days of indie sleaze. Which brings me to my next point: as well as waking up to the world of designer labels, throughout this next period our goth has become wise to the witchy wonders of self-care.

It may sound clichéd, but beauty is as much about feeling good as it is about looking good. And there's a whole world out there designed to make you feel good. This isn't about the pursuit of youth or perfection (more on this later) but rather of strength, health and vitality, both in the mental and physical sense. Maybe it's because there's so much stuff about death, ghosts and ghouls within the gothic canon, but there's a certain misconception about goths and their general approach to wellbeing. Being goth isn't about having a death wish, it's about drawing on a language of darkness as a way of arming yourself against the trials and tribulations ahead. It's about carving out a rigorous identity to help you navigate life's big uncertainties. Part of that requires mental and physical strength, which is where wellness comes in.

When you're young, you think you're invincible, but the older you get the more aware of your mortality you become. This is why now is the time to start taking care of yourself. So get a gym membership, go for a run, start journalling, switch off your phone, go outside, take time for yourself, meditate, say an affirmation, wear SPF, try a vitamin drip, get in a hyperbaric oxygen chamber, try cryotherapy, LED therapy, hit up an infrared sauna, get some essential oils, charge some crystals, put on a face mask, take your supplements, start hot yoga, cold yoga, room-temperature yoga, try pole dancing, join a Pilates class, eat well, sleep well, hydrate. Take pride in yourself and your body. But also have that glass of wine, eat that piece of cheese, order dessert, laugh, sleep in, stay out late, do something that scares you, and don't take life so seriously. Indulge the senses and whatever dark fantasies you may have. You don't need to become a vagina candle-burning, tonal knit-wearing slave to Goop. Indeed, wellness doesn't need to be perfect. It can be weird, messy and DIY, just as long as you are making some attempt at taking care of yourself, on your own terms. Because, ultimately, what could be more gothic than worshipping at the altar of the self?

BEAUTY CHECKLIST: THE ESSENTIALS

Just-bitten lips

The late Isabella Blow famously once said, 'If you don't wear lipstick, I can't talk to you.' A lipstick aficionado, she was never seen without a rouged pout, and even collaborated with MAC to create her own lip product. It's a similar story for sultry Spanish actress Rossy de Palma, who often offsets her strikingly angular features with a kohl-wrung eye and bold red lip. In fact, a signature of sepulchral sphinxes throughout the ages, nothing communicates dark glamour more than just-bitten lips.

Once viewed as a sign of wealth and status in ancient Mesopotamia, by the 16th century blood-red lips had become the hallmark of a fallen woman. It wasn't until the early 20th century that women were able to reclaim crimson pouts as a symbol of independence thanks to the suffragettes, who painted their lips scarlet as an act of sedition. The dual

connotations of power and transgression meant that by the
70s a bold red lip had become a vital component of the goth
aesthetic, and whether applied in matte, satin or lacquer, it
remains just as potent today.

Rouge nail polish

Picture one of cinema's most fabulously gothic vignettes:
Morticia Addams cutting the head off a red rose, her long,
spindly fingers accentuated by red lacquered nails that have
been sharpened to a sinister point. Laced with symbolism –
in ancient Egypt, only women of the highest-ranking order
were permitted to wear red – and just like a scarlet lip, nothing
communicates strength and power more than a red manicure.
Indeed, where chipped nails were the telltale trope of a young
goth coming to terms with herself, a meticulously applied coat
of crimson signals she's all grown up. Keep them classic in
ruby tones or lean into the darkness with rouge noir.

SPF

Vampires are by nature chthonic creatures: nightcrawlers
who draw their strength from darkness and burst into flames
at the first signs of daylight. Vampires are also fictional
creatures. But it does tie in nicely with goths who have similar
reputations for thriving at night. While they might not turn to
ash in sunlight, their skin will certainly endure irreversible
damage when exposed to it if left unprotected. Which is why
no beauty checklist is complete without a broad-spectrum
SPF. Buy it in a drugstore or get it from your favourite luxury
brand, just ensure it's above factor 30.

Crystals

Celebrated for their mystical powers and healing properties, humans have been using crystals in their ritualistic practices for centuries. The ancient Romans would carry tiger's eye talismans into battle as a means of protection. In the 12th century, Benedictine nun St Hildegard of Bingen wrote in the *Book of Gemstones* that onyx should be mixed into your drink to ward off illness. Meanwhile, according to feng shui tradition, amethysts can bring good luck in business. Fast-forward to today and you can buy water bottles containing selenite to combat burnout, cast spells on your ex or help manifest that sought-after promotion.

Whether you believe in the power of crystals or suspect them to be New Age woo-woo nonsense, simply having a crystal at home is a great reminder to start thinking proactively about your physical and mental well-being. Maybe a shiny piece of rock won't totally get rid of your midlife angst, but looking at it every day should certainly inspire you to make positive life changes that might go some way to alleviating all that bad juju. And there's something very comforting about that.

Yoga

Today, you'd be hard-pressed to find someone who didn't know their way around a downward dog pose, but in the 20th century yoga was still viewed as something strange, mysterious and even 'exotic'. While British sorcerer Aleister Crowley did nothing to dispel those attitudes, he did break down some of the rituals involved so that his followers could learn how to practise it. Published in 1939 by the Ordo Templi Orientis, Crowley's *Eight Lectures on Yoga* incorporated elements of astrology, science, mathematics, mysticism, Kabbalah and the ancient Indian practice of yoga, in which he became immersed at the turn of the century after travelling to Sri Lanka as part of his philosophical research. Crowley believed that the power to control your mind, and therefore the key to a higher state of consciousness and spiritual enlightenment, lay at the heart of this ancient practice. 'To train the mind to move with the maximum speed and energy, with the utmost possible accuracy in the chosen direction, and with the minimum of disturbance or friction. That is Magick,' he wrote. 'To stop the mind altogether. That is Yoga.'

Chapter VIII:
Gothic heroines, part II

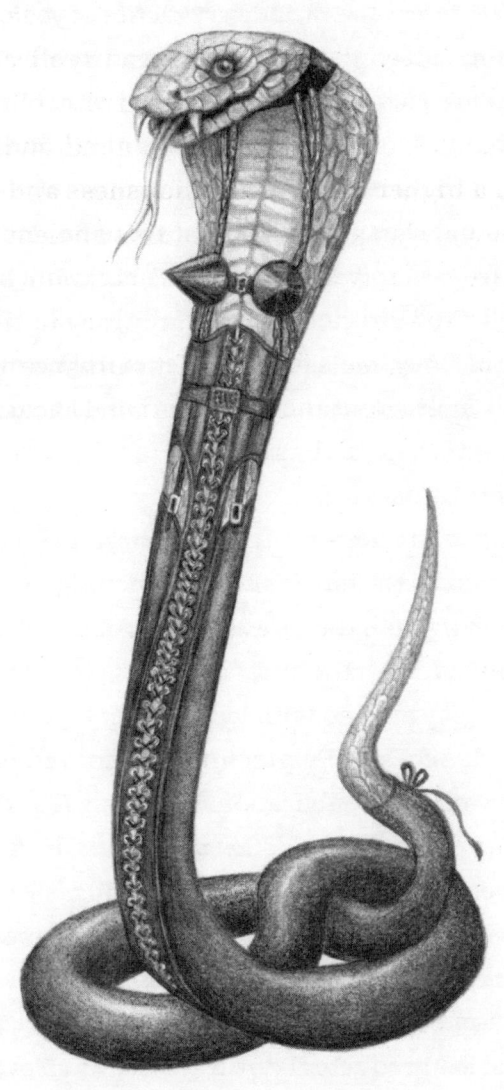

Katy England

Encountering Katy England's work is like falling down the rabbit hole. One of the fashion industry's leading stylists, she doesn't just create images, she creates whole worlds: upside-down, inside-out stories, whose characters have been plucked from fashion's rich subcultural history only to be chewed up and spat out as something entirely 'other'. Steeped in the language of the street, both past and present, she'll often blur the boundaries of gender or weave in an element of the perverse, from simply adding some lace to men's tailoring to putting actor and director Vincent Gallo in a pair of black hot pants and cowboy boots for the cover of *AnOther* magazine. The result feels spontaneous, emotive and punk – both beautiful and jarring at the same time, and always with some undercurrent of darkness.

Growing up in Cheshire in the 70s, England's sense of style was informed by the music she was listening to (Adam and the Ants, Spandau Ballet, David Bowie) and the nightclubs she frequented, with the latter providing the perfect arena in which to play around with looks. After studying fashion design at Manchester Polytechnic, she moved to London, where she worked at publications including *Elle*, the *London Evening Standard* and *Dazed & Confused*. It was during this time that she met Alexander McQueen, sparking one of the most important creative relationships the industry has seen.

From the first show she styled for him, The Birds in spring/summer 95, which was inspired by Alfred Hitchcock's 1963 thriller and featured actual tyre track marks all over models' bodies, to her work with him at Givenchy, England helped to define McQueen's raw and radical aesthetic. Remember that old 1998 issue of *Dazed & Confused*, which featured a cast of models with physical disabilities in custom-made designs by Hussein Chalayan and Rei Kawakubo and poked at the invisibility of disabled people in fashion? That was England. Highlighting the beauty of diverse bodies, she put double-amputee Paralympian Aimee Mullins in a wooden fan jacket by Givenchy and an antique whalebone crinoline, and styled model Sue Bramley, who is blind, in a beautiful butterfly mask by Philip Treacy.

Finding beauty in otherness is a theme that runs throughout her work, and it's something that informs her personal style too. Dressed in a palette of midnight hues, she often mixes 30s silhouettes with oversized tailoring, giving the otherwise image of faded grandeur a rock and roll twist, something that's accentuated by her smattering of tattoos.

Two other relationships are worth mentioning; one is with longtime collaborator Riccardo Tisci, another designer whose gothic sensibilities she has helped harness, particularly during his tenure at Givenchy, and the other is with her husband, Primal Scream frontman Bobby Gillespie, with whom she shares two incredibly gothic-looking sons, making them the ultimate modern-day Addams family.

Kembra Pfahler

Kembra Pfahler has worn many guises over the years: surfer chick, goth, dominatrix, punk rocker, filmmaker, artist, designer, model, muse. Above all, she is a provocateur, an explosion of monstrous female energy who once had her vagina sewn shut on film as a radical feminist statement.

Growing up in California during the 60s, she spent her youth catching waves on Hermosa Beach, but eventually swapped her sun-kissed life for the shadows after becoming obsessed with the dark women of horror movies. She moved to New York in the 80s to study at the School of Visual Arts and became immersed in the city's underground club scene shortly thereafter.

Drawing on the iconography of horror and German Expressionist cinema as well as Japanese Noh theatre, she formed a death rock band in the 90s called The Voluptuous Horror of Karen Black (named after the renowned American horror actress) which saw her and a troupe of twisted sisters transform into naked demonic figures with black ink-stained teeth, blood-red body paint, and towering bouffant wigs replete with crooked bows and thigh high lace-up PVC boots. It was during this time that she birthed a performance art movement she termed Availabilism, based on using whatever was available at any given time in her extreme and absurd performances.

Her work with the band informs much of her creative output as an artist, inspiring nightmarish prints and paintings based on her Mephistophelian alter ego, including painted imprints of her bum. She was also a huge proponent of the Cinema of Transgression, which saw her make love to a rubber octopus in Nick Zedd's experimental movie *War Is Menstrual Envy* (1992) in reaction to society's subjugation of women's bodies. Operating on the fringes of culture for most of her life, it's only in the last two decades that she's become embraced by the mainstream, having shown works at MoMA and the Whitney Museum.

Now in her 60s, she is just as bewitching as she was in her youth, perhaps now even more so, thanks to her trad-goth-meets-spooky-streetwear aesthetic and daring beauty choices: her long dark hair, the painted-on, almost vertical brows, dramatic rounded wings, and bold red or black lips – a look which has seen her model in recent years for brands including Calvin Klein, Rick Owens, Rodarte, Marc Jacobs, Mugler and Helmut Lang. Bold, extreme and goth to her bones, if you're ever experiencing a bout of self-doubt, just think: what would Kembra Pfahler do?

Kristen McMenamy

Kristen McMenamy's entire life has been underpinned by a refusal to fit in. An affront to orthodox ideas about beauty, she rose to fame in the 90s, thanks to her missing brows, translucent skin and androgynous, alien features. Here was a woman who once shaved part of her head just to stand out from other models.

Growing up in Pennsylvania, embracing her inner outsider always came naturally to McMenamy, which manifested visually through her extreme beauty choices. For example, she would often overline her lips in black and fill them in with white as a way to scare off bullies. It was only after seeing pictures of models in magazines that she realized she could turn her ridiculous limbs and awkward angles into a thing of beauty. So she put together a portfolio of images and set off for

New York. After a slew of initial rejections and suggestions (rebuffed, of course) to have cosmetic surgery, she got her big break in 1985 courtesy of Peter Lindbergh, who captured her quirks in a haunting campaign for Jil Sander.

Bucking the system once more, by the 90s she'd hacked off her long auburn locks, dyed the remains black and let makeup artist François Nars remove any shred of evidence of eyebrows. Suddenly she was everywhere. Fatigued by years of artifice and perfection, Amazonian bodies and supermodel good looks, it turned out that McMenamy's oddball aesthetic was exactly what the fashion doctor ordered. Rejecting the glamour and excess of the 80s, the industry had begun to turn in on itself; grunge was beginning to take off, heroin chic was beginning to creep in, and McMenamy became the face of the new world order.

Things continued this way throughout the 90s until she decided to take a break to focus on her family. She'd met the photographer Miles Aldridge in 1996 and married him in a fabulously high-fashion wedding, at which Karl Lagerfeld walked her down the aisle and Naomi Campbell acted as bridesmaid. Nearly a decade later, she made her return to the spotlight, this time with a shock of long silvery hair – because she simply couldn't be bothered to keep dying it. In an industry obsessed with youth, this was an act of defiance, the reverberations of which are still felt today.

Now in her 50s, McMenamy is as punk and rebellious as she's always been, which plays out daily via her Instagram account. After years of avoiding it (she was far too cool), a bout of lockdown ennui inspired her to download the app and she's been obsessed with it ever since. From her brash nude shots, outlandish outfits and Wednesday Addams braided pigtails to her incongruous backdrops (urinals/underground utility rooms), surreal props (dolls feature heavily) and confrontational notes of gore (a bloodied nose and a black eye – both from separate occasions), McMenamy's Instagram is the perfect antidote to the filtered vision of perfection we find clogging up our feeds. In short: she is an eternal reminder to be unapologetically yourself no matter what age you are.

Lily Munster

The idea for a show about a frightful family first arose in the 40s courtesy of acclaimed cartoonist Bob Clampett, who pitched it to Universal Studios. It wasn't until the 60s, however, when shows about housewives with secret powers and aliens living in the basement were gaining popularity, that the idea would be revisited. There was something in this domestic portrait of the supernatural that was clearly resonating with audiences: a spooky satire of the quintessential American family and their wholesome white-picketed fence life. And with that, *The Munsters* (1964–6) was born.

The 30s marked a golden age of horror for Universal, something the studio was keen to recreate for the small screen. And so, when it came to fleshing out the characters for a new show about a family of benevolent monsters, some 30 years later, they looked to their archive of iconic villains for inspiration. Herman, the family's benign but grotesque patriarch, is based on Frankenstein's dejected monster, while Sam Dracula, otherwise known as Grandpa, is cast in the image of Bram Stoker's creature of the night. Meanwhile Lily, who was brought to life by the scintillating screen siren Yvonne De Carlo, bears a strong resemblance to Frankenstein's bride.

A challenge to the stereotypical subjugated housewife archetype, Mrs Munster's domestic duties include using a vacuum cleaner to blow dirt around the house and further furnishing it with rubbish. Breaking convention and going against her husband's wishes, she experiments with various jobs, including as a welder, a palm reader and a model. At one point, she even opens her own beauty salon and tries to recreate disgruntled clientele in her own undead image. Simply put, she marches to the beat of her own funeral drum, something that manifests visually through her pale green skin, arched, angular brows, bold red lip and the vivid Mallen streak that lights up her otherwise ebony hair. As for her style, she's not like other ghouls, eschewing Morticia Addams's all-black aesthetic in favour of a pale pink paganesque gown.

The show only ran for two seasons, but every so often its characters are resurrected via various spin-off shows and feature films. Six decades on and with all her delightful eccentricities, Lily Munster remains an important fixture within the gothic canon.

Louise Bourgeois

Louise Bourgeois' work wouldn't go amiss in the Addams family house. Think of her gargantuan spider sculptures (1996–7) in all their monstrosity, or the hanging two-headed *Janus Fleuri* (1968) with its opposing male and female sexual elements. There's also *Avenza* (1968–9), the multiple-breasted garment fashioned out of latex and plaster that she's seen wearing in a famous photograph taken in 1975 by the photographer Peter Moor. Or the ominous, architectural *Cells* (1989–93) from which strange humanoid forms are suspended. Melancholic and macabre, Bourgeois' work deals with themes of loneliness, abandonment, female identity, family and fear, the last of which can be felt in the compulsive repetition of her key motifs: arachnids (which came to symbolize her mother, a weaver of tapestries and Bourgeois' first great protector), phalluses and labyrinthine lairs.

Born in Paris in 1911, Bourgeois' formative years were overshadowed by a series of traumas, including her mother's illness and eventual death and her father's various affairs – psychic phenomena that she would spend the rest of her life coming to terms with through her art. She was originally meant to study maths, but came to painting, printmaking and ultimately sculpture as a way of dealing with her feelings of isolation. Her work was largely put on hold during the 50s and 60s, during which she became immersed in psychoanalysis, emerging eventually with a new focus on organic sculptures with biomorphic bulges – the *Avenza* years.

Despite making her first ink-and-charcoal drawing of a spider in 1947, it would take another five decades for her to visit the subject again. In fact, some of her most famous and monumental spider sculptures were cast when she was 70 years old. Prolific right up to the very end, she died in 2010, one of the most important figures in modern and contemporary art.

Luisa Casati

In 1922, Surrealist artist Man Ray was photographing the esteemed Marchesa Luisa Casati when his electric lights burnt out the fuses at the Hotel du Rhin, leaving him with only the room's natural lighting. This, of course, meant a longer exposure, only the Marchesa was finding it impossible to hold still. The result is an eerie series of portraits that capture her in all her cadaverous beauty. One image, in particular, stands out; blurred from the double exposure, the Marchesa appears frantic and possessed, a ghostly apparition caught in between worlds. Staring straight out of the frame, she confronts the camera, her lips open like a wound, her eyes glassy and big like saucers, and her face flat like a mask.

The daughter of Milanese aristocrats who died when she was young, Casati was known throughout Europe for her decadent parties and outlandish behaviour. One story goes that she once gilded a servant in gold and ran through the streets naked carrying a crystal ball. She kept cheetahs on leashes and a boa constrictor in a glass case. Revered by the Surrealists and Futurists alike, she commissioned art, built palaces, practised sorcery, attended séances, read tarot and once went to the opera covered in the blood of a sacrificed chicken.

Six feet tall and emaciated like a human scythe, hers was a striking visage to behold, one of faded grandeur and decaying beauty. Cultivating this deadly image, she took doses of deadly nightshade to dilate her pupils and turn them black, ringed her eyes in kohl, caked her face in luminous white powder and dyed her hair a hazardous orange. She even fashioned fake eyelashes out of fabric.

Dressed by Poiret, Fortuny, Erté and Léon Bakst, her style was just as ostentatious; often draped in furs, feathers and veils, as she transformed herself into a work of living art. She even had a life-size doll made in her image, who she'd dress up and have seated next to her at the dinner table. Constantly trying to outdo herself, she ended her life in millions of pounds of debt, her homes lost, and her menagerie of wild animals all but dead. A constant muse, her legend lives on today through the work of designers from Karl Lagerfeld to John Galliano. And, of course, we'll always have those haunting images by Man Ray.

Lydia Lunch

According to legend, musician, spoken-word artist and general mischief-maker Lydia Lunch got her name from the makeshift meals she'd scavenge for Downtown's commune of struggling artists during the late 70s. A proponent of the no-wave scene, the New York post-punk music and art movement characterized by its abrasive noise and nihilistic worldview, Lunch has had many musical incarnations: the short-lived furore that was Teenage Jesus and the Jerks, whose songs featured lyrics like 'Little orphans running through the bloody snow'; Beirut Slump, 13.13, her solo artist era (during which she put out *Queen of Siam*, a clanging compilation of witchy songs); her 90s outfit Retrovirus and her most recent iteration, Big Sexy Noise, the moniker under which she still performs. But it was never really about the music. Her dissonant arrangements and piercing vocals are really just vehicles for her anarchic commentary, a way for her to dismantle taboos from female sexuality to suicide and sexual abuse.

A teen rebel (although she never really grew out of it), Lunch, whose real name is Lydia Anne Koch, grew up in Rochester, New York, and witnessed first-hand the rage that nearly tore the city apart during the 1964 race riots. This perhaps laid the groundwork for her own riotous energy, which she's been unleashing for the last five decades. It was that same fireball of female fury which saw avant-garde filmmaker Richard Kern cast her in two of his sexually transgressive films, *The Right Side of My Brain* (1985) and *Fingered* (1999) – both of which intensified her image as some kind of predatory seductress, eliciting both fear and lust at the same time, which she cultivated through her signature messy raven mane, blunt fringe, kohl-smudged eyes and raunchy all-black get up.

Now in her 60s, Lunch has lost none of her bite. In 2019, she released *So Real It Hurts*, a collection of barbed essays covering everything from environmental pollution to politics. She's also reinvented herself as a performance coach, hosted various female empowerment workshops, and is a successful podcaster. And she occasionally still performs her spoken-word poetry.

Lynn Yaeger

Lynn Yaeger is one of the most important fashion critics of her generation. She rose to fame in the 80s while working at cult New York newspaper *The Village Voice*, where she spent three decades penning an acerbic fashion column called Elements of Style. Instead of focusing on the clothes, she wrote about everything else, weaving searing social commentary, politically charged anecdotes and obscure historical detail into her reviews. When she did reference the clothes, however, she was never afraid to hold back, much to the chagrin of fellow industry pearl-clutchers.

This unconventional approach to fashion bleeds into her style, too. Born in Massapequa Park, Long Island, she realized early on that normcore dressing simply wasn't for her, swearing off trousers altogether – a principle she's abided by ever since. A magpie for vintage tutus and 20s pieces, her wardrobe has evolved over the years to include an eclectic mix of deconstructed Comme des Garçons, frothy Margiela tulle, antique crinolines, Victorian mourning jewellery, an assortment of Fair Isle cardigans and saccharine Simone Rocha confections – not to mention anything she might find rummaging around in a bargain bin.

As for beauty, her choices are even more daring. A cross between Betty Boop, Mamie Eisenhower and Louise Brooks, she's part 20s femme fatale, with her short, metallic russet bob and witchy micro fringe, and part cartoon pin-up with her rosy cheeks and exaggerated Cupid's bow pout. Victorian doll meets conceptual fashion Barbie, so iconic is her look that she has become something of a style muse for generations of designers and fashion insiders alike, particularly as she enters her later years.

Marina Abramović

According to internet conspiracy theories, Marina Abramović is a Satanic ring leader who eats dead babies for breakfast. While she does not worship the devil, she certainly has mystical powers, having cast a spell over the art world for the past five decades with her powerful, raw and sometimes violent work.

Born in 1946, in communist Belgrade, Abramović rose to fame in the 70s thanks to her daring performances, the most controversial and dangerous of which was *Rhythm 0* (1974). Spread over six hours, she offered up her body as a site of experimentation, where audience members were invited to do as they pleased with it, using a range of objects including a lipstick, paint, knife, whip, scalpel, chain and camera. It started gently, with members offering her a rose, until descending into chaos; her clothes were torn from her, her neck slashed, blood sucked and a loaded gun pointed at her head.

She left Serbia the following year after meeting her soulmate and creative partner, the German artist Ulay, with whom she spent the 80s working on performances that continued to test her thresholds of pain and endurance, in search of a higher consciousness and spiritual and emotional awakening. In 1988, after walking the length of the Great Wall of China, they decided to part ways, both romantically and professionally. It wasn't until 2010 that they would meet again, as part of Abramović's seminal performance *The Artist Is Present*, in which she sat in the Museum of Modern Art in silence for eight hours a day, over three months, while audience members sat opposite in individually allotted timeslots. One day she looks up and her face shifts from surprise, as Ulay takes his seat opposite her, to grief; the memory of a love long lost overcomes her, tears streak her face, and she reaches out to hold his now-old hands over the table. A breath, and her composure is slowly regained as the next audience member takes their seat a minute later.

During her career, she has lain both in the centre of a burning star and naked on a block of ice; she's deliberately rendered herself unconscious and held a bow and arrow directly over her heart. Moving in a new direction, her latest offering comes in the form of a film, in which she re-enacts seven iconic death scenes from the famous opera singer Maria Callas's stellar career, which is then screened alongside live recreations of Callas's most famous soprano arias from works by Bellini, Puccini and Verdi. Romantic, violent, bloody, beautiful, it's her most gothic piece to date.

From grandmother of performance art to grand high witch of wellness, in January 2024 she launched The Marina Abramović Longevity Method, a platform dedicated to sharing her experiences of various self-care practices and studies of ancient texts that she's accumulated over the years. It also sells her line of special tinctures that combine oriental, esoteric and traditional medicines to wicked effect.

Marjorie Cameron

The only redhead in her family, artist, actress and benevolent witch Marjorie Cameron Parsons Kimmel was born an outsider. Growing up in the Midwest during the late 20s, she spent her youth buried in art, poetry and magical thinking, the last of which she put into practice when she became immersed in the occult.

Cameron met her husband, the rocket scientist Jack Parsons, in LA after the Second World War. At the time, Parsons was living at the Agape Lodge, a US outpost of the Ordo Templi Orientis, a mysterious magical sect run by occultist Aleister Crowley. He'd been experimenting with Crowley's acolyte, L Ron Hubbard (he of the space lizards and Church of Scientology), on a ritual to conjure the Scarlet Woman or Babalon (the name given to powerful sorceresses in Crowley's preaching), when they suddenly came crashing into Cameron at a party. One look at her fiery red locks and he was hooked. But for Parsons, she was more than the incarnation of a Scarlet Woman: she was his Cinderella of the Wastelands, his Witch Woman, as he often referred to her.

Several years later, Parsons died in an unexplained explosion in his laboratory. Grieving, Cameron started to focus more on her art, producing a series of esoteric and erotic illustrations of angels, witches and strange demonic figures. Obsessed with 'blood rites' and black magic, she was dangerous and alluring. By this point, she'd chopped her hair off into a dramatic pixie cut replete with a witchy micro fringe, her elongated eyebrows were now pencilled in and she'd begun to waft around Hollywood in long ethereal robes. According to legend, she also drove around in a hearse – all of which led to controversial occultist auteur Kenneth Anger casting her as the Scarlet Woman in his psychedelic avant-garde film *The Inauguration of the Pleasure Dome* (1954).

A year later her work *Peyote Vision*, a hallucinatory drawing of a nude woman with a forked tongue being taken from behind by a sinewy creature, was published in the cult magazine *Semina*, triggering a police raid on the gallery where Cameron exhibited her art. Despite vowing to never show her work again, she has been featured in a handful of shows over the years, including at the Whitney Museum and the Centre Pompidou in Paris.

Cameron continued to make art and study astrology and the occult right up to her death in 1975, upon which her last Thelemite rites were carried out by a high priestess of the Ordo Templi Orientis.

Mary Shelley

Mary Wollstonecraft Godwin Shelley began writing *Frankenstein, or the Modern Prometheus* when she was 18 years old, after being challenged to a ghost-story writing competition by Lord Byron over a long and stormy weekend in Geneva in June 1816. Like her hapless protagonist, Shelley's life had up to that point also been marred by death. Her mother, the renowned feminist Mary Wollstonecraft, died shortly after giving birth, as did Shelley's new-born child, while her half-sister Fanny committed suicide some time later that year. It was out of this fraught psychic landscape that the seeds of Frankenstein, a story about a creature pieced together from cadavers – born essentially out of death – were first sewn. 'I saw the dull yellow eye of the creature open,' Victor Frankenstein observes chillingly of his creation before he abandons it. 'It breathed hard, and a convulsive motion agitated its limbs.'

In the absence of her mother, Shelley was raised by her father William Godwin, a radical philosopher and political writer. Though she had no formal education, Shelley would borrow books from her father's library and take them to her mother's grave, where she frequently went to read. She also spent her days writing letters, poems and short stories, publishing her first poem, 'Mounseer Nongtongpaw' in 1807. It was by her mother's grave that she was said to have conducted her affair with the married writer Percy Bysshe Shelley, who was a student of her father. Much to her father's chagrin, the couple eloped to Europe, which is when the infamous long weekend took place.

Published in 1818, *Frankenstein* is regarded as the first true piece of science fiction. Written during a period of enormous social change, when Enlightenment thinking – the progression of rational thinking and scientific advances – was being eclipsed by Romantic ideas about beauty, the sensory experience and the sublime power of the natural world, *Frankenstein* blurs the boundary between life and death, nature and nurture, good and evil.

Initially, people attributed the work to her husband, until Shelley published a revised edition under her own name in 1831. By this point, she had already been widowed (side note: despite being cremated on a beach, a piece of her husband's heart is thought to have survived, which Shelley had wrapped up in bits of his old poetry and shoved in a drawer for safekeeping). In a case of life imitating art, like her protagonist, she tried to distance herself from her own controversial creation. 'How I, then a young girl, came to think of, and to dilate upon, so very hideous an idea,' she wrote in the introduction to the new edition, before describing the story as coming to her in a dream. 'I saw—with shut eyes, but acute mental vision,—I saw the pale student of unhallowed arts kneeling beside the thing he had put together.'

Shelley wrote several other novels throughout her life, including *Valperga* (1823) and *The Last Man* (1826), about a lone survivor of a terrible plague. Echoing the latter, Shelley was herself the last woman standing, having lost every family member by the time of her death in 1851. But like our other gothic heroines, her legacy as one of the literary world's most brilliant minds remains just as commanding, if not more so, today.

Michèle Lamy

Michèle Lamy has lived many lives: defence lawyer, boxer, artist, activist, political rebel, sorceress, cabaret dancer, designer and restaurateur. Mutating from one to the next, her seven decades on this planet have been shrouded in mystery, something she cultivates through her own avid storytelling. Like a mirage, every time you think you have arrived at some kind of truth about her, it vanishes into thin air.

What we do know, however, is that she was born in the Jura region of France, in 1944, where she was sent to a Catholic boarding school from a young age, the constraints of which she found, unsurprisingly, quite challenging. Law came first, then cabaret, until eventually she decided to up sticks in 1979 and move to LA, where she set up two of Hollywood's most exclusive hotspots: Café des Artistes and Les Deux Cafés, the latter of which was staged in a car park and frequented by the likes of Joni Mitchell, Madonna and Sharon Stone.

It was in the early noughties in California that Lamy met the designer Rick Owens, her very own prince of darkness, who lovingly refers to his paramour as Hun – in reference to the barbarian ruler Attila the Hun, that is, rather than a cute abbreviation of 'honey'. For the past three decades the formidable duo have been serving up their stygian brand of glamour and dystopian vision of the future under the OWENSCORP banner, which makes everything from clothes and accessories to beautiful brutalist furniture. Beyond that, what Lamy is really good at is building worlds, something she does under her personal banner Lamyland. Take the *Bargenale*, the scaffolding-entombed barge that served as a restaurant, hang out and floating recording studio that she created for the 2015 Venice Biennale. Or *What Are We Fighting For*, the immersive boxing gym she built in London's Selfridges in 2018.

Lamy is one of those rare entities who embodies both artist and muse, a mindset that extends to her physical appearance and singular vision of beauty. There's the diamond- and gold-encrusted teeth, the tattooed fingers, the smear of black on her forehead, the artfully distressed hennaed hair and the signature eyes encircled with kohl. Her approach to style is equally arresting. Weathering the waxing and waning of trends, Lamy's all-black uniform consists almost exclusively of Comme des Garçons and Rick Owens creations, distorting her petite frame with their exaggerated proportions. In a world full of imitators and clones, Lamy is uniquely her own, which is what makes her so alluring.

Chapter IX:
The goths and goth-coded:
in their words, part II

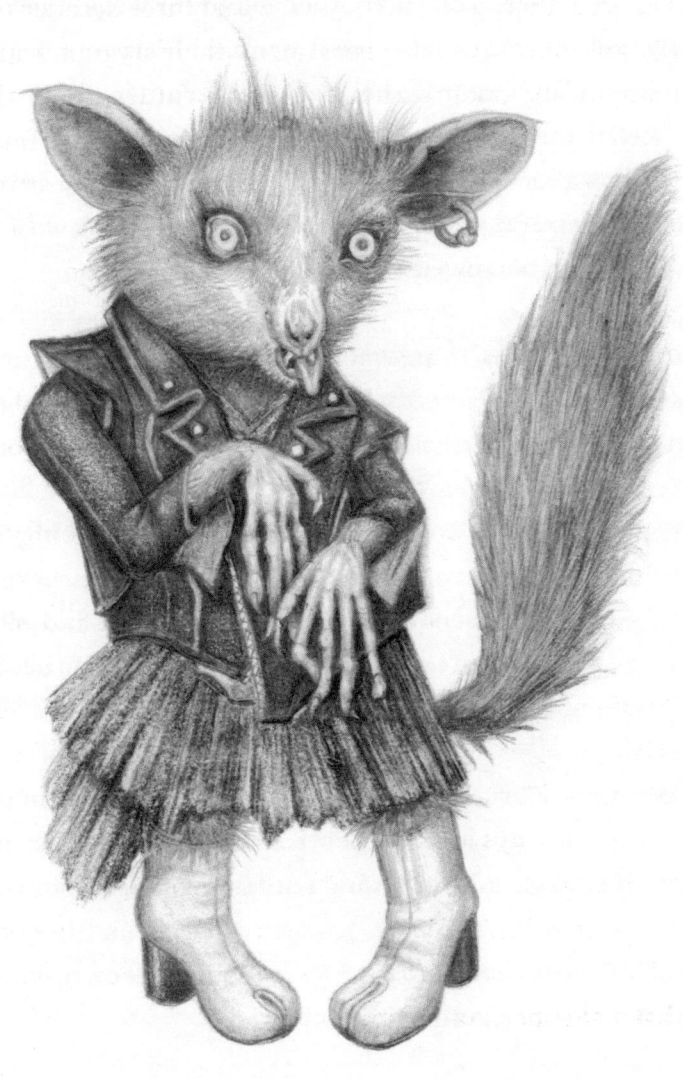

Devon Ross, musician, model and actress

'I guess I always sympathized and related to rebels in a way. I feel more comfortable and myself with black hair. Whenever I have to dye it another colour for work, I never really feel myself until I dye it back. Sid Vicious, Dave Vanian and Suzi Quatro in her black leather jumpsuit always appealed to me.

'Goth is a form of expression, I guess. I can't say I ever classified myself as a goth, but whether I was conscious of it or not I've always borrowed a few things from the goths.'

Dilara Findikoglu, designer

'Real goths don't call themselves goths. Even in the 80s, they didn't call themselves that. In 2024, I don't define myself as one thing, but I am drawn to the romance, poetry and storytelling of the goth aesthetic. To me, goths represent a community of like-minded people.

'I always tend to wonder about the unknown, the dark side of things, what we can't see, which is why I'm drawn to black. It's mysterious. Most of the things we see as darkness are just part of life.

'With my work, I'm trying to give lightness through darkness. I always look for depth. Behind the harsh look, there's always some emotion and sensitivity.'

Gabbriette Bechtel, model

'Goth is something you can't define.'

Holli Smith, hair stylist

'120 Minutes on MTV was an alternative and goth music segment that blew my mind when I was growing up, and gave me exposure to the idea of self-expression and identity. It matched the feeling I had not understood inside. Complex and confusing. Grey and nothingness took over in life at times. Empty and dark but there is something in even this space that exists.

'The goth aesthetic matched what I was trying to understand inside. A goth aesthetic was the non-category category. It was not mainstream. It was new, and naturally, it aligned for me to be drawn into this. I found protection in the expression. Others saw on the outside of me for once what I was feeling inside without words. Only a few were drawn but the right people saw that there was a comradery in what I was flagging. It seemed to put people off actually but that was part of the resistance to being a normative, judgemental and homogenized human. I wanted the mystery. I wanted the unknown. The strength of this was the beginning of my strength today.'

Inge Grognard, makeup artist

'I think I was born with the spirit of goth inside. What was at first a bit of a struggle with the establishment around me gave me the strength to become the makeup artist I am now. I projected my world, attractions and feelings onto faces and images in our house, and being with somebody who is similar-minded made it even stronger. It gave me peace with my inner self. Now I would call it dark romanticism.'

Isamaya Ffrench, makeup artist

'I've always felt quite style-less. For the most part, I like to dress for functionality; if I can't run 10K in a pair of shoes, I don't feel excited about wearing them. My friend once said the best way to dress consistently with your character is to pick three words that describe your style and make sure every time you choose an outfit, you hit all three words. For me, they are 'practical', 'gothic' and 'ancestral'.

'I'm often drawn to masculine aesthetics and struggle with feeling too outwardly feminine. I feel like the gothic genre is the perfect interplay of masculinity and femininity. There is something both romantic and courageous about it. It has intensity and exudes an intellect that other styles don't. Perhaps this is because it's synonymous with the Romantic period, writers like Percy Shelley, John Keats and Lord Byron for example, or the metal music genre, which is arguably one of the most musically complex and intellectual genres. The gothic style allows you to embody and connect to these classical touchpoints, ultimately allowing you to 'be' and associate symbolically to intellect, depth and romance.'

Josephine Lee, aka Princess Gollum, model and artist

'As humans we go through lots of phases, shedding layers as we evolve but at the core we mostly remain the same, kind of like stars. I'm not sure why I am drawn to all things black. I love wearing jewellery or pieces of clothing that can physically hurt me, and listening to music that all my friends think is sad. I find it to be soothing. I didn't really choose this, it really is just what comes naturally to me. Sometimes I feel luminescent inside on a gloomy day. Light doesn't shine half as bright without darkness. There's something calming about the fact that there is another side to the coin for pure joy.

'Goth is always cunt in my world. When I was in grade school and discovered the goth/emo styles, I thought it was about the way you dressed, the way you pounded on lighter shades of foundation from the drugstore and how much eyeliner you could pack on. Throughout the evolution of life, I realized that it's not about the clothes you wear at all. I could be in a full pink monochromatic look but still look, feel and be goth. It's a mindset, an energy, from the core. It's acknowledging the darkness that exists, finding the beauty in it and honouring it. Goth bitch 'til the day I die.'

Katy England, stylist

'While I don't present myself as gothic as such, I make choices in dressing which allow me to play with my different personalities. I like to combine the masculine and feminine, and while I lean towards the darker, less palatable side, I like to add some romance to soften out its edges. There is no doubt that my attraction to the darker side is so instinctive, so primal that I wonder where it all began. Does our aesthetic seep into each cell through generations past or did it emerge when I first opened my eyes and saw my pale-skinned, black-haired, dark-eyed mother and father? The magnetism of darkness is a powerful one.

'Black, the root of gothic, is so calm and confident. Quiet, yet it speaks volumes. I share the great Yohji Yamamoto's opinion, who has been working almost exclusively in black since his beginning. "Black is modest and arrogant at the same time. Black is lazy and easy – but mysterious. But above all black says this: 'I don't bother you – don't bother me'." For the curious, that's not only intriguing but there's also a danger involved. It's unknown, so can stimulate an intrepid desire to unpeel the dark exterior, which a "true" goth has purposefully constructed referencing imagery around death. Like watching a horror movie, it evokes fear and thus adrenaline to fuel the attraction.

'Constructing clothing or making outfits in all black reduces silhouette and shape to its purest form. Eliminating the voice of colour allows real focus. Adding detail or decoration with only black textures is a delightful journey into the possibilities of light, dark, soft, rough, shiny, sheer, stiff or fluid, and so on. It can be so sophisticated, escaping all seasonal trends and undoubtedly remaining the favourite colour of the fashion industry.'

Kembra Pfahler, artist

'For me, the term goth, clearly and obviously, represents the other side of lightness, which is darkness. I would say that darkness and blackness represent every colour and everything. Whereas light or whiteness is only one thing. So goth-ness is an adventure. The opposite of beige.

'What appeals to me about a darker aesthetic is it gives me the courage to look into the sun. Like the camera obscura, which I learned about from the filmmaker Kenneth Anger. What I love about the darker aesthetic is that it's encouraged me to never want to stop learning.

'I'm from Los Angeles, California, the antithesis of what goth culture might be about. I grew up where everyone wore bikinis, surfed and lived in the sunshine. I gravitated towards gothic culture and goth-ness through the Universal horror films, and through black-and-white films. My heroes of the gothic culture in this country have been people like Charles Addams and Don Bachardy, who was Christopher Isherwood's lover. I loved his drawings so much. It was so funny to me because he always used to draw people so intensely that I saw real beauty in his ugliness.

'I would describe my style as being someone who makes use of what is available. I gravitate towards contrarianism, and my favourite style is to wear what no one else wants to wear. I'd like to be the poster child for unwanted style. My beauty choices are made at age 62 living in New York City, as wanting to dress and feel as beautiful as I can be on any given day. I don't dress to impress, I'm not dressing for someone else's approval. The impetus for me being an artist is trying to look for beauty where there is none.'

Kristen McMenamy, model

'Goth means to me rebellion, about saying "fuck you" to mediocrity. It's about standing aside from the pretty norm, being bold, being dark and eternally rebellious. Undead chic!

'I would describe my style as being or trying to be an extension of my inner feelings. I always keep an element of the gothic. I never want to be too ladylike or likewise too masculine. I like a bit of androgyny, a bit of eccentricity and always a bit of obtrusiveness. And my number one rule: big dark sunglasses.

'For beauty, I love a black smokey eye and white skin. If I have makeup on, I like to leave on the eyes so that in the morning I have a messed-up, hungover-looking look. It adds an element of danger and darkness. Especially in the morning Pilates class! I also like to wear my eyes nude with white skin and a big blood-stained red mouth.'

Chapter X:
Ageing goth:
notes on style

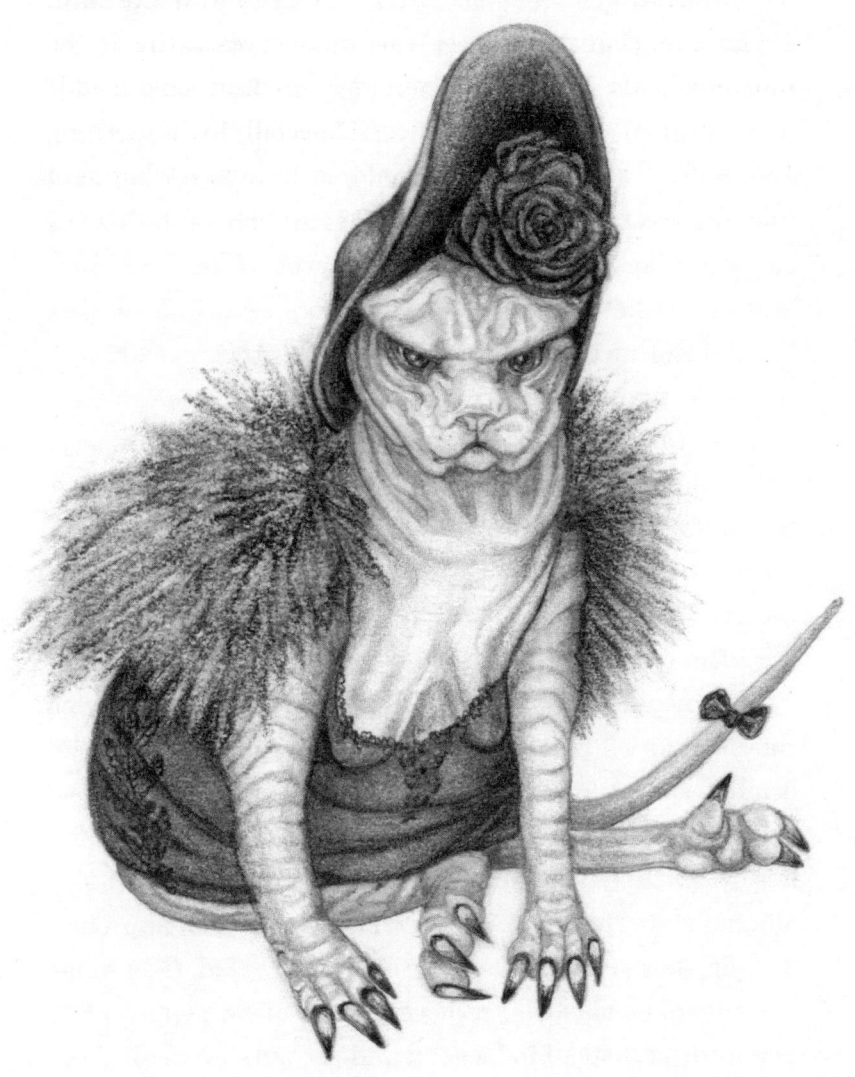

As the twentieth-century poet Edith Sitwell famously once remarked, 'Good taste is the worst vice ever invented.' She also lamented on another occasion that 'the trouble with most English women is that they will dress as if they had been a mouse in a previous incarnation; they do not want to attract attention.' Sitwell was certainly no mouse. Bucking the conservative conventions of the day, she fashioned herself into one of Britain's most esteemed eccentrics, becoming even more outlandish as she aged thanks to her sculptural turbans, exotic plumes, gold collars and rings the size of saucers. Like Sitwell, Marjorie Cameron's flare for drama only intensified with age; the artist and occultist swanned around Hollywood in the 50s and 60s draped in exquisite robes like a nomadic sorceress.

Fast-forward to the rare birds of the 21st century: octogenarian Michèle Lamy is a nightmarish vision in tentacled Rick Owens padded down; Helena Bonham Carter channels a vampy sex appeal in Vivienne Westwood; the grand high art goth Marina Abramovic´ has replaced her utilitarian clothing of old with high glam gowns; you might spy performance artist Kembra Pfahler in a Mugler catsuit or an all-black Adidas tracksuit. And of course, the original sphinx Siouxsie Sioux continues to thumb her nose at tradition with her trad goth latex body suits (designed for her by Scottish designer Pam Hogg – the duo have had an alliance since the 80s). Although singular in their approach to style, these women have one common thread: they rebut the unspoken sartorial codes expected of women over 50, demanding instead to be seen and recognized in all their brilliant eccentricity. And they do that through the saturnine language of goth.

Let's not beat around the greying bush here. There is – sadly – still an expectation for women to become increasingly invisible as they age. You've done your bit and now you're excused. Please make way for the newer, younger, perkier, less wrinkled, less burnt-out and less jaded model.

But the insurgent spirit of goth runs in your lifeblood; withering into the abyss of old age with a nice cardigan (unless it's ironic) is simply not an option. Instead, as you enter this next phase of womanhood, it is time to go bigger, badder and bolder than ever before. Indeed, to be goth in your twilight years is to take up even more room, whether that's with gigantic proportions, dramatic silhouettes, extreme layering, unusual fabrics or outrageous accessories. It's about being cavalier in the face of good taste and wearing whatever it is that makes you feel good. With age comes a certain sense of freedom and a 'don't give a fuck' attitude that you've flirted with for most of your life, but are only now at a point where it finally feels authentically yours. There's no more rampant imposter syndrome to navigate, or sartorial codes of conduct to adhere to – not that you were particularly good at that anyway. You are now free to be totally who you are.

If, when you're young, style is a projection of who you want to be, in these later years it's a reflection of who you actually are; the culmination of various iterations of self in the life-long search for identity. By the time you've clawed your way here, there's nothing left to prove. You've hurled your way through menopause, midlife crises and various mental breakdowns. You've changed careers, houses, boroughs, sexual partners, friends, tax brackets, accountants, doctors, politics and sexual partners again. You've managed to put your kids (if you have them) through school and come to terms with their resentment/embarrassment/general hatred of you. Maybe you've been made redundant at some point, retired, gone through a divorce, endured extramarital affairs, partaken in them – or maybe you're still single. Wait, there's more: by now your posture is fucked, you're as grey as a badger, your eyesight is fading, you can't pull on a winklepicker without groaning, gravity is winning, the war over whether to go under the knife or not rages on, and death is ever looming. It's certainly claimed a few of your loved ones already. The silver lining to this dark cloud is that you can now ride the bus for free!

They say youth is wasted on the young, which is partly true. During the one period in your life where you have all this energy and curiosity about the world without any real responsibility, you're crippled by a self-consciousness that prohibits you from truly expressing yourself. By the time you've entered those final witchy winters, however, that self-consciousness has fallen away. Only now you're weary and disillusioned. The world has also moved on and is obsessed with the next best (read: young) thing, and you're just expected to wilt away until there's nothing left of you. But personal style is a journey. If you arrived fully formed in your youth, unfettered by teen angst or a desire to grow, change, and become something truly great, it would take away both your drive for, and the fun of, self-discovery. And besides, expressing yourself in outlandish and outrageous ways at a time when you're expected to simply shrink from visibility is the most subversive thing you can do.

So what exactly does this third and final phase hold for you sartorially? Anything really: the world is your oyster. Lean into your eccentricities, go futuristic and architectural or indulge in ostentatious displays of grandeur. Reference the clubs of your youth, or mix trad goth with the codes of the modern-day street. Add a splash of colour for a dissident distinction. Go full Lolita goth or go home. The whole point here is to surrender to total freedom of expression and fearlessly embrace your authentic self.

STYLE CHECKLIST: THE ESSENTIALS

Rick Owens's down

Rick Owens was making puffer jackets well before he started collaborating with Moncler. But since their first joint collection in 2020 – a monstrous reimagination of the Italian outerwear brand's padded down through Owens's sinister lens – his puffers have become something of a staple. Extreme and futuristic, the collection comprised strange asymmetric forms with billowing tentacles and funnel necks, rendered in Brobdingnagian proportions. There were sleeveless tunics, cropped jackets and large coats with elongated sleeves all in jet-black and supernatural silver. Striking a balance between function and flamboyance, comfort and discomfort, it was first introduced to the world via a specially made tour bus that Owens had lined in padded down. The next time they collaborated was for the brand's 70th birthday, for which Owens refashioned Moncler's iconic Maya jacket, adding his signature architectural lines, girded shoulders and gauntlet-like sleeves. The poster girl for both collections was Owens's wife, Michèle Lamy, for whom these twisted quilted creations have become a kind of second skin, adding exaggerated form to her otherwise diminutive figure. A must for any ageing goth, simply throw it on for your weekly supermarket trip and push that shopping trolley in style.

Fur

Humans have been wearing pelage to protect themselves from the elements for as long as they've existed, but it wasn't until ancient Egyptian times that fur, particularly leopard skin, became a symbol of social status for both emperors and high priests alike.

The Marchesa Casati was said to have a whole wardrobe full of exotic pelts and fur-trimmed cloaks. She also used to take her pet cheetahs on midnight strolls around the Venetian piazza where she lived wearing nothing but a shaggy coat and pearls. Write that down. In fact, there's a wonderfully gothic painting of her by the artist Augustus John in the National Museum, Cardiff, painted in 1942, 15 years before her death, in which she appears enveloped by a voluptuous black stole, her signature kohl-wrung eyes hidden behind a funereal veil, while a black cat sits menacingly upon her lap.

Louise Bourgeois is another gothic heroine who constantly shrouded herself in fur during her later years. In an iconic photograph of the artist by Robert Mapplethorpe, taken in 1982, she's seen grinning at the camera in a dark tufted coat, while clutching one of her giant phallus sculptures, *Fillette* (1968). In another series, taken by Belgian-born photographer Alex Van Gelder, she's shown sitting on a chair encased in a sumptuous white pelage, with a blanket on her knee.

There's something inadvertently perverse and fetishistic, in the Freudian sense, about wearing fur. It both elevates its wearer and reveals their base, animalistic side; the id to your ego. It calls to mind the Surrealist artist Méret Oppenheim's *Object* (1936), a hirsute teacup that scandalized Paris when it was first introduced, due to its connotations of displaced female sexual desire and lesbianism. Venus in furs. A staple for the ageing goth, fur can be worn on any occasion and in any style, whether it's a full-length coat or simply fur-lined, or even as a standalone collar thrown over the shoulders at the last minute. That said, it's important to note: any fur that adorns your gothic body must be vintage or faux. We're not in the business of mindlessly slaying animals, here.

Comme des Garçons tailoring

Wearing a piece of Comme des Garçons tailoring can sometimes feel like an assault on the body, in the near annihilation of its natural form. But it's also strangely empowering. Like Rick Owens, designer Rei Kawakubo subverts the codes of femininity to create something unsettling, exquisite and totally unique. Using a mix of ruffles, tubing, origami-like folds and sprouting cascades of fabric, she magics into being these bloated bulbous forms and biomorphic shapes, sometimes monstrous and gigantic and at other times fragile, like some delicate cocoon. Take her spring/summer 2016 collection, titled Blue Witches, which was an expression of dark female energy in opera coat form. This wasn't the first time Kawakubo had taken inspiration from the occult. Her autumn/winter 2004 collection was even witchier, with its roots in Victorian mourning dress. Think deconstructed leg-of-mutton sleeves and pleated taffeta bustles. Ideal for your grand high witch era. For the full effect, try to get your hands on some vintage Comme, but if you're looking for something a little more restrained you can always find something more recent.

Vivienne Westwood corsetry

Vivienne Westwood wasn't a goth – she was very specifically a punk – but she had gothic sensibilities. Let's call her an honorary goth. Fiercely independent, she did things on her own terms, and was always diametrically opposed to the establishment. She was also drawn to macabre symbols, often using skulls and bones in her work as well as bondage elements like harnesses and chains, which is all very elementary goth-in-training stuff. A far more interesting proposition, however, for women in this third stage is her corsetry and other garments of that ilk. Steeped in romanticism, historicism and a dark witchy energy, it's empowering to see an older woman with a cinched-in waist and sweetheart neckline, a powerful celebration of her feminine allure. It doesn't have to be a corset in the traditional sense, either. What Westwood was so great at was creating garments that have an element of corsetry, whether that's one of her gathered poplin frocks with its basque waistline, crepe bustier tops or an off-the-shoulder corset cardigan, the kind of thing you'd imagine Morticia Addams would start wearing after the kids have grown up and left home. Just look at Helena Bonham Carter or London DJ Princess Julia, both of whom ooze gothic glamour whenever they wear Westwood. And it's incredibly versatile – you can dress it down with an ironic Fair Isle cardigan or jazz it up with a vintage fur stole and some pearls, and you have yourself an achingly eccentric outfit.

Streetwear

The only truly modern way to dress is eclectic, mixing and matching your style periods and codes. There's a lot here about fur, jewels and corsets, which pertain to a very specific idea of old-world glamour, grandeur and femininity. This is where the avant-gardism of Comme des Garçons tailoring and the monstrosity of Rick Owens down come in, as a necessary means of contrast. But there needs to be another element, a palate cleanser to all that opulence. Something intellectually a bit lighter and more pop. Enter: full-look Adidas tracksuits, oversized tees, shrunken hoodies, hooded vests, ironic Juicy Couture velour, tight Lycra, Y-3 trainers and notes of denim – naturally, all in black. It's what Kembra Pfahler does so well, pairing Rick Owens with trad goth textures (latex, net and leather) and the language of the street in the form of T-shirts, hoodies, jeans and boiler suits. In fact, Pfahler recently collaborated with Rick Owens on a drop of stygian streetwear, comprising trucker shorts, jumbo tees, tank tops, stocking boots and chunky high-top sneakers, all of which bear the logo of her band The Voluptuous Horror of Karen Black.

The wedding dress

Throughout her rule, Queen Victoria made two major stylistic contributions to the gothic tradition. One was the strict black Victorian mourning dress, and the other was wedding whites. Before her day, brides would dress in a variety of hues, with red being the most popular. Bucking tradition in her usual fashion, for her wedding to Prince Albert in 1840 she wore an ivory silk-satin gown with festoons of bobbin lace lining the neck and sleeves. It was such a spectacle that the style immediately spread throughout Europe, with white being imbued with connotations of purity and innocence.

Back then, it was typical for women to wear their wedding dress on numerous occasions. Someone who took this to the extreme was Charles Dickens's deliciously gothic anti-heroine Miss Havisham, who was so consumed by the trauma of being jilted by her fiancé on the morning of her wedding that she never took her gown off again, spending the rest of her days a nightmarish vision in phantom white. Since then, the image of an ageing woman in a decaying wedding dress has been enshrined within the gothic canon. Instead of purity and innocence, it's come to signify something altogether macabre. It calls to mind another gothic heroine: the titular character from Tim Burton's *Corpse Bride* (2005), another tragic Victorian figure hellbent on revenge. Today, wearing full-look bridal whites to anything other than your own wedding is an act of sedition worthy of the boldest of goths. Indeed, by emancipating the wedding dress from its traditional context, and its association with the perfect, demure virgin woman, it is the ultimate affront to the establishment.

It's a look that Marina Abramović has championed over the years. For her harrowing *Balkan Baroque* performance, as part of the 1997 Venice Biennale, she sat atop an altar of bloody cow bones, shrouded in marital whites; for her final cycle of *The Artist is Present* performances, she wore a long chantilly cream gown with a high neck and wide train; and in 2020, as part of her *7 Deaths of Maria Callas*, she commissioned Riccardo Tisci to create her an exquisitely ethereal ecru lace wedding dress.

But this doesn't mean you need to hit up your local bridal boutique. Instead, look for festive elements that you can incorporate in your arsenal: cobweb-like lace, smokey swathes of tulle, infinite layers of ruffles. Lean into the romanticism with Simone Rocha cream broderie anglaise; sex it up with an off-white, off-the-shoulder Vivienne Westwood draped Ginnie dress; indulge in the ghostliness of it all with a 30s satin gown. Or go conceptual with a piece from Comme des Garçons's autumn/winter 2005 Broken Bride collection and kill two birds with one stone.

Hats

In his 1954 *Little Dictionary of Fashion*, Christian Dior wrote: 'Without hats there is no civilization.' Women have been wearing head coverings since ancient Egyptian times as a way to protect themselves from the outside elements and to demarcate social status. In the Middle Ages, they were encouraged to wear them to cover their hair as a sign of virtue and modesty, whereas today headgear is an expression of individual style and identity.

Wearing a gigantic or opulent hat indoors feels incredibly punk – look at Katharine Hepburn's net and feather confection in Tennessee Williams's Southern Gothic *Suddenly Last Summer* (1959). It also prevents people from constantly looking over your shoulder, which always comes in handy at social events. Nobody seemed to grasp this quite so effectively as Dame Edith Sitwell. Adding height and flourish to her already eccentric look, hats became something of a signature for her, particularly in her later years. To celebrate her 75th birthday, she commissioned a series of portraits by society photographer Cecil Beaton, in which she can be seen in a selection of flamboyant head coverings, each one more extravagant than the last. Particularly alluring is a black organza turban and a cap with coq feathers and tulle that fans out like a peacock's tail.

Isabella Blow was another major fan of fine headpieces, whether in the form of giant antlers, a phosphorescent perspex disc or barbed wire fashioned out of feathers. So legendary was her love of hats that she was even buried in one: her favourite pheasant fascinator by Philip Treacy.

Extravagant jewels

The Marchesa Casati once famously declared 'I want to be a work of art'. She spent her life trying to be exactly that, adorning herself in jewels – crosses, pearls and strange wire creations – that she had specially commissioned from the greatest designers and artists of the period. As legend has it, she once anaesthetized a snake, leafed it in gold and wore it to a dinner party as a necklace. Because who hasn't been tempted to do this?

Where crucifixes and ankhs are the telltale semaphores of youth, these days our goth has graduated to more substantial adornment. Case in point: granny pearls. Where no self-respecting teenage witch would be caught dead in a string of pearls, let alone several, now that she's in her third phase of womanhood nothing could be chicer. Because, by this point in your life, you've cultivated such an eldritch aesthetic and outsider identity that wearing something so traditional is actually quite subversive. It's the same for granny cardigans and black Chanel tweed (see Amanda Harlech). Besides, pearls are a symbol of wisdom, which, if nothing else, you now have in bucket loads.

An important note here: don't break the bank on precious fine jewellery; instead opt for vintage costume pieces and keep your eyes peeled for cheap thrills while on your travels.

NOTES ON BEAUTY

So often, the state of being goth is associated with the idea of eternal youth, what with all that talk of vampirism and the undead. On the contrary: ingrained in the goth psyche is a staunch refusal to submit to restrictive ideas about beauty, so nothing could be more goth than embracing the visible signs of age, such as wrinkles, sun spots and maybe a whiskery mole. That's the theory, anyway. And it's partly true, but it's also a bit more complicated than that. If I wanted to neatly and succinctly wrap up the argument I've been making throughout this entire book, which is that being goth is all about sticking two fingers up to the establishment and celebrating your authentic self just as you are, I would tell you at all costs to put the needle down and step away from the knife, before listing all of the gothic women I admire who would rather stick pins in their eyes than Botox in their face. But it's not as clear-cut as that. For starters, I work in the beauty industry, which means I've already stared down the point of a needle. Curiosity got the better of me. But more importantly, and this is also what I've been arguing throughout these chapters, is that being goth is about doing whatever the fuck you want, no matter what anyone says; wearing whatever you want to wear and looking however you want to look, whether that's as if you've driven through a wind tunnel or like the back end of a Shar-Pei. When it comes to beauty and personal appearance, the only person whose opinion matters is yours.

There is, without a doubt, a misogynist societal pressure placed upon women to defy the ageing process, no matter how painful or expensive, while men are generally speaking free to go about as they please without fear of being replaced romantically or professionally by a younger model. Instead of buckling to this pressure, as women and goths we should feel empowered in our decision to greet old age like an old friend. After all, there is so much beauty in a face etched with experience, where each crevice tells a story of a life well lived and where every laugh and smile can be mapped out. But in the same breath, there shouldn't be any stigma in wanting to preserve the face you've come to know and love (it might not have always been that way) for as long as humanly possible. If you want to make a Faustian pact with a doctor on Harley Street, you should be able to do exactly that without any shame attached. It doesn't make you any less of a goth. Who hasn't seen the highly camp and wonderfully macabre *Death Becomes Her* (1992) and not wanted to drink the Isabella Rossellini Kool-aid? Or felt a tingle of excitement at the thought of Patrick Bateman's psychotic self-care routine? And there's nothing wrong with that (although admittedly neither of these stories end particularly well). It's only when people start lying about the various procedures they've had done that we get into murky waters. Shame has no business in the world of goth.

It's the same with hair. There's an expectation that women should start dyeing their manes at the first signs of greying, to which the obvious goth response would be: go fuck yourself, which is exactly what model Kristen McMenamy did when her hair started to blanche in her late 30s. With her long white witch locks, she's almost more beautiful, more ethereal now than she was in her youth.

But embracing your greys isn't a prerequisite to the goth condition. Just look at Princess Julia, no wave provocateur Lydia Lunch, or fearless agitator Cosey Fanni Tutti, all of whom have kept their eldritch locks intact. There's also designer Pam Hogg, who bucks convention with her acid-yellow hues, and fashion critic Lynn Yaeger with her signature crop of livid red hair.

Once again, when it comes to makeup, there is no single way of expressing yourself. Much in the same way you'd approach style in this period, there's something to be said for taking things to the extreme. Take Yaeger's doll-like rosy cheeks and accentuated Cupid's bow (the childlike nature of which calls to mind Bette Davis's exquisite gothic heroine Jane Hudson in *Whatever Happened to Baby Jane?* (1962)). But you can also do away with makeup altogether. The point is you should be able to do whatever it is that you want with your appearance as you sail into this final period, without giving two hoots about what people think. You've come too far to turn back now.

BEAUTY CHECKLIST: THE ESSENTIALS

Grills

Forget the image of a pair of false teeth floating in a glass of water, for ageing goths its all about grills. Humans have been furnishing their teeth with jewels and precious metals for centuries. It all started with the Etruscans, who would lavishly wrap their teeth with gold wiring, not just to hold replacements in place, but also as a means of communicating wealth and status. It's a similar principle to that adopted by hip-hop legends of the noughties, for whom blinged-out grills became something of a style phenomenon. When Jermaine Dupri announced, 'We about to start an epidemic with this one,' at the beginning of Nelly's 2005 music video for 'Grillz', he wasn't joking. Augmented smiles have become a symbol of power, individualism and otherness, particularly for women of a certain age, because it's completely unexpected. Consider Michèle Lamy's diamond dentures or Erykah Badu's glinting grin. In equal parts hypnotizing and horrifying, grills, tooth gems or other dental ornamentation are the perfect witchy addition for any ageing goth.

The signature cut

Rei Kawakubo has maintained her sharp, jaw-grazing bob and boxy fringe since she was a student. It's the same for Lydia Lunch, whose chaotic raven locks and choppy bangs are almost Samson-esque: change these, and you take away some of her power. Where youth is a time of exploration and experimentation, these later years are all about reflecting who you are, and the easiest way to convey that is with a signature cut. Having something that announces your presence before you even open your mouth, something unmistakably unique to you is a great way of communicating power and prowess. It also shows that you are not afraid to be who you are.

Black eyeliner

When it comes to being goth, copious amounts of black eyeliner will never go out of style, no matter how old you are. It's dark, it's dramatic and, to paraphrase that wise old sage Yohji Yamamoto, it says: 'I don't bother you – don't bother me.' Which is exactly what you want at this point in your life: not to be bothered. The great thing about black eyeliner is that there are myriad ways to wear it, whether that's a feline flick, smudged in the water line or smeared haphazardly onto the lid. For added drama, you can create almost-vertical ovoid wings like Kembra Pfahler to accompany your near-vertical drawn-on brows.

Horns

During the 90s, the French artist and provocateur Orlan (she of mononym fame) underwent a series of plastic surgery procedures as a way of reclaiming her body from the clutches of the male gaze. Using her own flesh as a raw material, she emerged from one operation with a pair of demonic implants inserted just above the brow line as a challenge to normative ideas of beauty. So bewitched by the barbaric beauty of this artistic expression was the Belgian designer Walter Van Beirendonck that he based the beauty look for his autumn/winter 1998 collection on Orlan and her mutant bumps. Now in her 70s, she's just as outrageous as ever, often accentuating what she refers to as her 'lumps' with silver eyeshadow and glitter. Vivienne Westwood, our honourary goth, was another proponent of horns, which she used to wear on a hairband that the brand still sells today – far less of a commitment than going under the knife, yet equally subversive in its allusions to the devil.

Hair dye

Reaching for a bottle of hazardous-looking hair dye can feel just as invigorating during this later phase as it did during those teen tearaway moments. Forget the bubblegum-pink and powder-blue rinses synonymous with stereotypical grannies – this is about vivid red, lurid yellow and even radioactive orange. Or if you really want to scare the mainstream, opt for two-tone black-and-white in the style of Orlan.

Dark lips

Where a bold red lip might have seen you through your various midlife crises, as you enter this next phase it's time to dial up the drama with more stygian hues. Indeed, nothing communicates dark glamour more than a deep black lip. Yes, it's liable to leave a noticeable calling card on the neck or collar of any young lover, but pair it with a dark oil-slick eye and you'll probably scare them off anyway.

Chapter XI:
Gothic heroines, part III

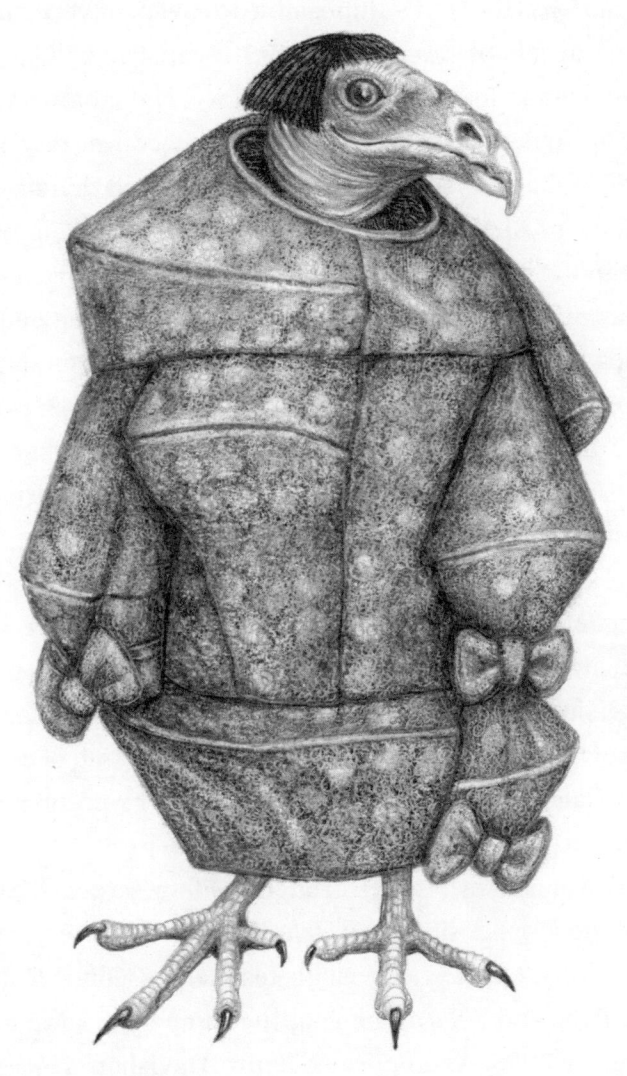

Miss Havisham

Miss Havisham is Charles Dickens's mad, bad ageing bride and the main antagonist of his famous novel *Great Expectations* (1861). It's impossible to escape if you studied English at school, but if not, a quick recap: Once a beautiful young woman lost in the throes of love, Havisham's whole life is upturned when she is jilted on her wedding day by the dastardly Compeyson. Unable to move beyond this singular tragic event, she haunts the halls of her crumbling mansion like a living ghost. Surrounded by decay, her life remains a shrine to this one moment; she stays dressed in her wedding clothes, now eroded with time; the clocks have been stopped at twenty minutes to nine, the exact moment she learned that Compeyson wasn't coming; the wedding feast, now rotten, is still laid out on a table, and a single unworn shoe remains exactly where she left it. Consumed by revenge, she adopts a young ward named Estella and trains her to be cold and cruel, to encourage men's affections and then rebuke them, starting with Pip, the novel's protagonist. In true Dickensian style, by the end of the novel Havisham sees the error of her ways and seeks to make amends but, of course, it is too late, and she dies tragically after her wedding dress catches fire.

Miss Havisham has been brought to life on screen countless times, most hypnotically by Helena Bonham Carter in Mike Newell's 2012 film, and most grotesquely by Olivia Colman in the BBC and FX's spine-tingling romp of an adaptation, released in 2023. A complicated figure, Havisham's inclusion in this list is not to extol the virtues of seeking revenge on the entirety of the male population, but rather to hold her up as an example of an older woman completely self-possessed; here is someone who defies the conventions of her age by her sheer visibility, and she does it by drawing unapologetically on the aesthetic of goth.

Morticia Addams

Morticia Addams is the macabre matriarch of that creepy and kooky, mysterious and spooky cast of characters created by cartoonist Charles Addams in 1938. A satire of the archetypal 20th-century American family, and a response to the cultural malady that was sweeping the nation in the time of the Great Depression, the Addamses are a strange aristocratic tribe who delight in all things deviant and unnatural.

Morticia, whose name derives from the Latin word 'mort', which means death, is a diabolical vixen whose family descends from a long line of Salem witches. Madly in love with her husband, Gomez, she uses torture as a form of foreplay and spends her free time frequenting séances, chopping off the heads of flowers and nurturing her garden of deadly nightshade. She's fiercely loyal and protective of her children, and yet paradoxically encourages them to run with scissors. She is smart and intelligent, has a wicked sense of humour and unorthodox worldview, coming up with lines such as: 'Normal is an illusion. What is normal for the spider is chaos for the fly', and – my favourite – 'Embrace your darkness, for it is what sets you apart.' In short, she's not like other ghouls, and she isn't afraid to show it.

An inky apparition, Addams is always represented as the embodiment of gothic glamour, dressed in a jet-black bias-cut dress with tentacles along the hem and sleeves. Her skin is marble-like and deathly and her hair is long and raven-hued. Her eyes are either kohl-ringed and heavy or elegant with a simple feline flick, and her lips are rendered in crimson or rouge noir. Over the years, she has been brought to life by a sling of deadly beauties including Carolyn Jones in the 1964 television series and Anjelica Huston in Barry Sonnenfeld's *The Addams Family* (1991) and its 1993 sequel.

'Morticia is elegant, glamorous and humorous,' says Huston. 'Fern Buchner, Kevin Haney and Ruth Myers were responsible for her overall look. Ruth Myers had a very clear view of how to combine beautiful, striking and scary to create such an iconic character. Then it was up to me to personify her and bring this otherworldly figure to life.'

The ultimate dark siren, she's been influencing goths to simply be themselves since her inception, and will continue to do so for generations to come.

Patricia Morrison

Patricia Morrison has been in more bands than you can shake a drum stick at. Lending her black magic and sepulchral charm to each one, she is one of goth's true mavericks, and one of the few female artists to succeed in a largely male-dominated space. Growing up in California, Morrison started playing bass as a teenager, inspired by the glitter and glam of artists such as Roxy Music and David Bowie. She formed her first band, Femme Fatale, in 1975 along with Alice Armendariz; it later morphed into Masque Era. In 1977, their musical landscape exploded after attending their first punk gig, and they promptly formed The Bags, a punk band with an all-female line-up who inexplicably all wore bags on their head while on stage.

Morrison spent the late 70s and early 80s pogoing from band to band before eventually being drawn to the shadows of goth. Now living in London, she started touring with Siouxsie and the Banshees as part of Fur Bible, before joining goth crooners The Sisters of Mercy. Rattling bones with her spooky aesthetic – her long inky locks, luminous skin, high arched brows, kohl-rimmed eyes and haemoglobin-hued lips, not to mention the Victoriana-meets-sex-shop get-up – she was the perfect addition to frontman Andrew Eldritch's eerie ensemble. So enamoured was he by Morrison that he wrote 'Lucretia My Reflection' about her, in which he compares her to Lucrezia Borgia, the Renaissance noblewoman notorious for her rumoured love of poison. Things eventually turned sour, and Morrison left the band in 1989 to become a motorcycle courier.

In 1996, she returned to music to join forces with the harbingers of darkness The Damned, marrying morbid frontman Dave Vanian in Las Vegas that same year. After touring with the band for several years and giving birth to her daughter Emily, in 2005 Morrison finally hung up her winklepickers and spiked dog collar. But her legacy lives on through her generous contributions to goth music and style.

Poison Ivy

Kristy Marlana Wallace was walking down the street in 1972 looking for a ride home when fellow Sacramento College student Erick Lee Purkhiser pulled up alongside her. He'd spotted her on campus from a mile off with her crimson corkscrew curls, halterneck top and hot pants with a hole in them that exposed a gash of red panties underneath. The next time they met was in an Art and Shamanism class, when Purkhiser went and sat beside her – a meeting that would ultimately change their lives and the face of music as we know it.

Better known as Poison Ivy and Lux Interior (inspired by an old Coasters song, the name came to her during a magic mushroom trip, while he took his from an automobile advert) these two lovebirds were the driving force behind psychobilly band The Cramps. Founded in 1976, with Bryan Gregory on second guitar and Pam Ballam on drums, the band staged their first performance at New York's legendary punk club CBGB. Interior was writhing on the floor, deep-throating the microphone, while Ivy was firing her guitar – a rare Canadian model – as if it was a rifle. Ivy was working as a dominatrix at the time, and so was dressed head to toe in vinyl, a look that later evolved to include garter belts, animal print onesies, sequined bras, belly dancer skirts, a prom-queen tiara, Bettie Paige bangs and Egyptian-queen kohled eyes. Sure, she was a flame-hot pin-up, but she was also so much more than that. Her skill at the guitar was positively demonic – and she was largely self-taught.

Born in San Bernardino, California, Ivy was always a bit of a miscreant; smoking in the girls' loos at school and generally making mischief. Her parents moved around a lot, so music was her only constant. She'd mess around on her brother's guitar, but it wasn't until she saw Bo Diddley's *Sacramento Live* in the early 70s, during which he performed with a female guitarist named The Duchess dressed in gold lamé, that she realized music was something she could pursue.

The Cramps was a band for outsiders, rulebreakers and displaced misfits. Exploring the macabre side of mid-century Americana, with references to budget B-movies and horror comics, their songs conjured potent images of eyeballs in martinis, human flies, Jayne Mansfield's near-decapitated head, alligator men and teen werewolves, while their sped-up, psychotic brand of 50s rockabilly and oogie-boogie voodoo sounds spawned an entire sub-genre of music.

They continued to rattle bones until Interior died in 2009, forcing Ivy to retire from music. But her memory as one of the most formidable women in rock and roll's history will forever haunt us.

Simone Rocha

For over a decade, Irish designer Simone Rocha has been changing the way we think about femininity. Though she draws on traditional feminine motifs (think: frothy tulle confections, festooned with flowers, ribbons and bows), there's always an underlying tension that lurks beneath the surface; an interplay between toughness and fragility, comfort and unease. Her autumn/winter 2021 collection was an ode to the schoolgirl goth. Pretty on the outskirts, a latent edge ran throughout, as gossamer-fine tulle spilled out of cropped leather biker jackets and platform combat boots were adorned with pearls.

She's also influenced by nature, ancient religious rituals and twisted Irish fairy tales. For her autumn/winter 2022 collection, she was inspired by the Irish legend of the Children of Lir, a sinister tale about four children who were turned into swans by a jealous stepmother. Against the saturnine backdrop of a medieval hall in London, models morphed into cygnets with knitted balaclavas and winged skirts, while black overcoats with billowing sleeves harked back to Victorian mourning dress.

A walking billboard for her eldritch aesthetic, Rocha's own look is very specific; she wears almost exclusively head-to-toe black, almost always in one or several of her own creations, her long dark hair piled effortlessly up onto her head. The people who she designs for are also very specific. Arty, ethereal types who eschew trends and normative ideas about beauty and who are often drawn to the macabre; in short, the modern goth.

The daughter of Chinese-Irish designer John Rocha and his creative partner Odette, Rocha grew up in Dublin. At first, she tried to resist a career in the family business, opting instead to study art at Dublin's National College of Art and Design but, as it turned out, fashion was the only language through which she could truly express herself. She moved to London to study at Central Saint Martins and set up her own eponymous label in 2010 upon graduation. A slew of accolades and awards followed; she was a finalist for the LVMH Young Fashion

Designer Prize in 2013 and won her first British Fashion Award for Emerging Talent a year later, graduating to Best British Womenswear Designer in 2016 and eventually Best Independent British Brand in 2021.

Fast-forward to today and Rocha has worked on lucrative collaborations for J Brand, Moncler and H&M, has stores across London, New York and Taipei, and is arguably one of the brightest stars showing on the London Fashion Week calendar. And she does it all on her own terms.

Siouxsie Sioux

Siouxsie Sioux's contribution to the gothic canon cannot be underestimated. In fact, the modern goth might not even exist if it wasn't for this dark temptress; it certainly wouldn't have had such an enduring impact on culture. The irony is that Sioux would recoil from any such association with the movement.

Born Susan Janet Ballion, even her upbringing could be described as gothic: her father was a scientist who was said to milk snakes for venom and who died when Sioux was just a teen. A self-identified outlier, she paints her childhood in suburban Chislehurst as being incredibly lonely. This acute sense of otherness is what drew her to the burgeoning punk scene, and she quickly became one of its most notorious proponents. So inflammatory were her sartorial choices that in 1976 she was attacked at a Sex Pistols gig for wearing a cupless latex bra and matching suspenders, a pair of fishnet tights and a Nazi swastika armband. That same year, she put together the first iteration of what would eventually become Siouxsie Sioux and the Banshees, which took its name from the Vincent Price-helmed horror movie *Cry of the Banshee* (1970), and convinced Pistols manager Malcolm McLaren to let them perform at the 100 Club Punk Festival, during which she gave a howling 20-minute rendition of 'The Lord's Prayer'.

The first incarnation of the band featured boyfriend and long-time collaborator Steven Severin, who had only picked up his first guitar a day earlier, drummer Marco Pirroni and notorious renegade Sid Vicious. It was Severin who directed the band's sinister sounds, often referencing Krautrock bands such as Can, Kraftwerk and Neu!, as well as composer Bernard Herrmann, particularly the screeching strings he created for the famous shower scene in Alfred Hitchcock's *Psycho* (1960), while Sioux composed the band's harrowing lyrics, which she would grab sporadically from newspaper clippings.

By 1978, the new line-up consisted of Sioux, Severin, John McKay and Kenny Morris, and the band put out their first single, 'Hong Kong Garden', having signed with music label Polydor that same year. By this point, punk had started to wither and the shadow of goth began to loom. Three months after 'Hong Kong Garden' reached number seven in the UK singles chart, the band put out their debut LP *The Scream*, which would ultimately become recognized as one of the first true gothic albums.

Throughout the 80s and 90s, both their line-up and musical landscape shifted, but the band lost none of their mesmerizing and moody charm, particularly in the case of

Sioux, whose haunting beauty and unique approach to style had become the stuff of legend, having ditched the extreme shock tactics of punk in favour of a much more dark but romantic aesthetic. In fact, her Cleopatra-style eye makeup and hair like a blackbird's nest, not to mention her hardcore fetishistic get-up, would inspire legions of copycats for years to come, much to her chagrin.

Though the band eventually parted ways in 1996, and her side project The Creatures with band member Peter 'Budgie' Clarke, wrapped up several years later, Sioux's reputation as one of music, and indeed fashion's, most hypnotizing individuals will endure forevermore. Her recent sold-out solo performances throughout the UK is a testament to that.

Susie Cave

With her porcelain skin, coal hair and glittering emerald green eyes, Susie Cave's beauty is otherworldly. Wraith-like and romantic, she floats through time and space like some ethereal being. In the 2014 film *20,000 Days On Earth*, her husband, post-punk's Prince of Darkness Nick Cave, describes their first encounter as a hallucinatory experience. 'All the endless, impossible fantasies, the young girls at the Wangaratta pool lying on the hot concrete, Courbet's *Origin Of The World*, Bataille's bowl of milk, Jean Simmons's nose ring, all the stuff I had heard and seen and read . . . Caroline Jones dying in Elvis's arms, Jackie O in mourning, Tinkerbell trapped in the drawer, all the continuing, never-ending drip feed of erotic data came together at that moment in one great big crash bang and I was lost to her and that was that.'

Growing up in Cheshire, Cave's ascent to stardom is the stuff of fashion legend. Desperate to escape the strict conventionality of her British boarding school, she stole away on a milk float in search of a better life. She was just a teenager when she was scouted to be a model and quickly became muse to a host of photographers (Helmut Newton, David Bailey and Guy Bourdin) designers (Azzedine Alaïa, Vivienne Westwood and John Galliano) and musicians (Prince, Bryan Ferry and ultimately Nick Cave) alike.

The pair married in 1999 in a medieval chapel and welcomed twin boys shortly afterwards. They spent the next decade tucked away in a seafront Regency house overlooking the Brighton Pier, complete with a Pepto Bismol-pink kitchen and unexpectedly quaint façade. It's these surreally twee and hyper-feminine elements which make the whole thing so deliciously gothic.

In 2014, Cave returned to the spotlight with the launch of her label The Vampire's Wife, named after one of her husband's unfinished novels. A collection of 30s-inspired dresses, vintage-looking separates and cloaks rendered in rich velvets and luminous lamé, the brand is Cave to the core. In fact, her aesthetic is so distinctive that the women who wear her designs, such as Keira Knightley, Florence Welch, Ruth Negga and Liberty Ross, look like they belong to a strange and beautiful cult, where members dance around stone circles and mutter incantations under moonlight. From cult label to industry stalwart, with her gothic twist on the hyper-feminine, nearly a decade on from its inception, Cave's powers are only getting stronger.

Rossy de Palma

Spanish actress and gothic muse Rossy de Palma has spent her life turning tradition on its head. Born in 1964, she moved to Madrid in the 80s, where she became immersed in La Movida Madrileña, a counter-cultural revolution that emerged after the death of fascist dictator Francisco Franco. It was around this time that she met acclaimed director Pedro Almodóvar, who came to see one of her hypnotic performances as part of the leather-clad pop punk band Peor Impossible. So captivated was he by her DIY glamour that he offered her a part in his film *Law of Desire* (1987), on the condition that she dressed herself and did her own makeup, which at the time was steeped in the lurid hues of John Waters's transgressive cinema. Marking the birth of a close creative partnership, over the past four decades the pair have worked together on eight films, including masterpieces like *Women on the Verge of a Nervous Breakdown* (1988), *Tie Me Up! Tie Me Down!* (1989), *Broken Embraces* (2009) and, most recently, *Parallel Mothers* (2021) about the Spanish Civil War and a jarring maternal mishap.

Despite initially being dismissed by the Spanish media because of her unconventional looks (with her strikingly angular features, she's a cross between a Modigliani and Picasso painting made flesh), throughout her career she broke down barriers and redefined what a movie star could look like. And then she did the same for modelling, after catching the eye of designers Jean Paul Gaultier, Thierry Mugler and Alexander McQueen, who cast her in many of their shows.

Inspired to make other women feel as confident in their own skin, in 2017 she launched a line of beauty products with MAC inspired by her favourite Surrealist artists.

Now in her sixth decade, she continues to inspire designers, artists, directors and photographers alike with her flamboyant style (note the fans, turbans and exotic plumes) and signature beauty choices (lashings of kohl and a distinctive crimson pout) – so much so that she was recently tapped to star in Saint Laurent's autumn/winter 23 campaign.

Rei Kawakubo

Rei Kawakubo is one of the most influential women in fashion. With her avant-garde designs she has taught us to question the very notion of what fashion is. And yet she herself is a complete enigma. Fiercely private, the very few interviews she grants raise more questions than they answer. The closest she's ever come to explaining herself was with the title for her spring/summer 2014 collection, which was 'Not Making Clothes': because Kawakubo doesn't make clothes, she creates concepts. And for this collection in particular, those concepts were brought to life through a riot of padded cages and mutant bulbous forms, a rubber ring suspended on chains and a neon-pink teddy bear that spilled out of confetti-like frills.

Born in Tokyo in 1942, Kawakubo left home in the 60s, back when clothes were still just clothes. But the impulse to cut and paste and remix was beginning to take shape, and she began work as a stylist, often customizing garments or fabricating entirely new ones. She was 27 when she launched

Comme des Garçons, the banner under which she began propagating her signature aesthetic: asymmetric black silhouettes that have come to form the basis of most self-respecting goth's and/or fashion editor's armoury.

In English, Comme des Garçons translates as 'like some boys', but Kawakubo could never be accused of being like anyone, a fact that was brought into sharp relief when she unveiled her brand in Paris Fashion Week in 1981. By this point, business was booming in Japan, where she had well over 100 stores, but was largely unknown in the West. Meanwhile, in Paris the industry was ablaze with glamour, colour, opulence, sex, sequins and rhinestones, epitomized by the work of Thierry Mugler and Gianni Versace. No one could have predicted the revolution Kawakubo was about to start.

Picking at accepted ideas of beauty, femininity and even taste, each show has been more mind-blowing than the last. Over the years, her strict uniform of black has given way to elements of colour, but her precision when it comes to form remains unchanged. Four decades on, and the brand has evolved into an empire. There's the colony of global stores and franchises, and the cult collaborations with Nike. There are all the diffusion lines and the lucrative perfume business. There is Dover Street Market, the cultural behemoth and conceptual department store which Kawakubo redesigns each season. There was the 2017 retrospective at the Met. And then there are the fans: legions of devoted fans who worship at the altar of fashion's longest-serving deity. All. Hail. Rei.

Wednesday Addams

Named after a line in the famous children's nursery rhyme about Wednesday's child being full of woe, Wednesday Addams is the delectably droll daughter of Gomez and Morticia Addams. Though first conceived in the 30s as one of Charles Addams's illustrations, she was brought to life in 1964 in a TV adaptation of the comic series, played by actress Lisa Loring. But it was Christina Ricci's immortalization of the fledgling goth in Sonnenfeld's *The Addams Family* (1991) and its sequel, which remains ingrained in popular consciousness. Indeed, from her acerbic one-liners to her apathetic stare, Ricci's incarnation as Addams struck a chord with oddballs everywhere.

Dressed in a black tea dress with a Peter Pan collar and with her hair worn in plaited pigtails, her childish exterior belies something much more sinister within. Here is a girl who delights in all things grim and grotesque, and who spends her days hanging out in graveyards, torturing her brother, and just generally plotting world obliteration. 'Come, sorrow, we welcome thee,' she declares in *Addams Family Values* (1993). 'Let us join in grief, rejoice in despair, and honour the fortunate dead.'

'Young girls are traditionally supposed to be pleasing and to behave,' says Ricci. 'And with Wednesday, here is a young girl who is so self-possessed that she absolutely refuses to behave in any way that isn't 100% true to who she is and how she feels. How a person expresses themselves aesthetically follows through with who they are inside. Being so self-possessed and refusing to pander to anybody else, Wednesday dresses herself in a very unique way. I think all of that really appealed to people who felt that they have never been allowed to be themselves and have always felt the pressure to be pleasing, or other than who they really are inside.'

Three decades on and the character has been resurrected by Tim Burton in the Netflix series *Wednesday* (2022–). Played by Jenna Ortega, cinema's reigning scream queen, this most recent iteration of Addams is her most dynamic and nuanced yet. The show follows the maudlin teen as she starts her first term at Nevermore Academy (note the Edgar Allan Poe reference), a school for outcasts, monsters and freaks, where she struggles with complex relationships, both new and old, romantic and familial, and burgeoning supernatural powers. An allegory for teenage rebellion, it's no wonder the show holds the record for most hours (over 300 million) viewed in a week for an English-language series. Season two remains hotly anticipated as a result.

Winona Ryder

From her agitated performances to her salty off-screen antics, if there was one person who could encapsulate the coming-of-age goth experience it would be American actress Winona Ryder. Where other Gen X starlets were perky and toothy-smiled, Ryder was awkward and cool, wide-eyed and mordacious. She cut her hair short and wore vintage clothing in mostly midnight hues; read J D Salinger and dated skinny pale boys like Johnny Depp; she spoke publicly about feeling lonely and turned eye-rolling into an art form.

Born in Minnesota, Ryder grew up in a commune in California, where she'd watch old movies against a barn wall. Her first role was that of tomboy Rina in David Seltzer's coming-of-age drama *Lucas* (1986). But it was as Lydia Deetz in Tim Burton's seminal goth flick *Beetlejuice* (1988), the disaffected teen obsessed with death and dressed permanently as if in mourning, that made her a household name.

In *Heathers* (1988), Ryder's performance as the monocle-wearing cynic Veronica Sawyer, whose extreme bout of schoolgirl ennui pushes her onto a path of violence, is a biting portrayal of what it's like to be young, goth and frustrated. In *Mermaids* (1990) she plays the misunderstood misanthrope Charlotte, who dresses head to toe in black and spends the entire film wrestling her devout religious views and disdain for her promiscuous mother with her own burgeoning sexual desires. In Francis Ford Coppola's *Dracula* (1992), she lives out the ultimate gothic fantasy as Mina Harker, Count Dracula's virgin bride; and in *Girl, Interrupted* (1999) she plays Susanna Kaysen, the morose 18-year-old who ends up in a mental hospital after chasing a few aspirin with a generous slosh of vodka. Ryder's next move will see her reprise the role of Lydia Deetz, who's now all grown up, in the hotly anticipated Tim Burton *Beetlejuice* (2024) reboot.

Ever since her 80s and 90s heyday, throughout her early noughties fall from grace (those all-black court 'fits were nothing but iconic) and right up to her recent revival as the 2022 face of Marc Jacobs, and through her recurring role as the frenzied Joyce in cult sci-fi drama *Stranger Things* (2016–),

Ryder has remained a beacon for misfits and melancholics around the world.

Theda Bara

The gothic aesthetic owes a lot to 20s screen siren Theda Bara. Coming of age during a time when studio bosses were first realizing the potential of star power, both on and off screen, cinema's leading ladies were typically given beguiling backstories. Bara, for example, whose name was an anagram of 'Arab death', was said to be either the daughter of a French actress and an Italian sculptor, or a Middle Eastern potentate, born miraculously in the shadow of the Sphinx. In reality, Theodosia Goodman was the daughter of a Jewish tailor who grew up in Cincinnati. Nevertheless, the press were keen to fuel studio rumours further, describing Bara as being the reincarnation of historical femme fatale Elizabeth Báthory, a Hungarian countess and alleged serial killer, and the equally murderous Lucrezia Borgia.

Bara further cultivated this sense of dark exoticism by holding press conferences in hotel suites that had been transformed to look like Middle Eastern harems, with tiger skin rugs draped over the floor. Shrouded in incense and surrounded by arcane artefacts, Bara would bewitch her audience with tales about ancient Egypt and the occult. Like the costumes she wore on film, her outfits had a timeless and 'exotic' quality about them; she wore mysterious veils whenever she went outside, while her robes were low-cut, gauzy and revealing, often accentuating her voluptuous curves. She would also wear crowns, bangles and big hoop earrings, and carried a gold cigarette holder. In a marked departure from the classic bob favoured by the reigning flappers of the period, Bara wore her hair long and unruly, while her makeup was inspired by acclaimed Polish makeup artist Helena Rubinstein, who encouraged Bara to emphasize her eyes with graphic wings, lashings of mascara and kohl eyeliner in a nod to the original sphinx, Cleopatra, along with overlined, angular brows. This she wore with chalky white foundation and bold red lipstick.

A veritable sex symbol, Bara is credited with creating a new female archetype: the stygian seductress who would flaunt her sexual charms for nefarious purposes. This was in no small part due to the characters she inhabited on screen, in particular the role of an unnamed vampire in the silent movie, *A Fool There Was* (1915), in which she mimes the immortal line, 'Kiss me, my fool!'

Throughout her career, she made over 40 motion pictures, in which she played variations on this idea of a heartless temptress, which is what ultimately earned her the nickname 'Vamp'. By 1919, Bara's star had begun to fade, and she was eclipsed by clean-cut actresses like Clara Bow and Louise Brooks. However, seven decades on from her death, Bara remains an important cultural icon for generations to come.

Vampira

Morticia walked so that Vampira could float. Finnish-American actress Maila Nurmi was attending a costume ball in Hollywood in the 50s as Charles Addams's morbid matriarch when she caught the attention of Hunt Stromberg Jr, a big-time TV producer who was so hypnotized by her vampiric allure that he invited her to host a series of late-night fright films in the guise of her gothic alter-ego, whom she christened Vampira. Airing on KABC-TV from 1954 to 55 and on KHJ-TV from 1955 to 56, *The Vampira Show* was a huge success, and propelled the aspiring actress and model to stardom.

Shown draped over a chaise longue, stroking her pet spider, or bathing seductively in a cauldron, Nurmi captivated audiences with her dark sense of humour and signature spine-tingling scream. Her set was camp and theatrical, shrouded in smoke and scattered with pumpkins, cobwebs, skulls and other Halloween ephemera. She oozed sex appeal; where Morticia was cadaverous, Vampira was sultry and curvaceous, a Jessica Rabbit type, or perhaps her evil twin. Nurmi drew on elements of bondage and the burlesque that she took from John Willie's *Bizarre* magazine and the bewitching pin-up Bettie Page. Her look was always the same: an extreme cinched-in waist, plunging neckline and glamorous wiggle skirt, seamed stockings and fishnet tights. Meanwhile, her approach to beauty was just as dramatic, from the extreme arches of her drawn-on eyebrows, to the beauty spot on her cheek and her sharp blood-clot claws.

For Nurmi, Vampira wasn't just a role, she was a vital part of the actress's artistic expression – so much so that when she refused to sell the rights to her hallmark character, the show was promptly cancelled. Her next big appearance came courtesy of *Plan 9 From Outer Space* (1957), the doomed science fiction film about gravediggers, ghouls and flying saucers, directed by cult filmmaker Ed Wood and featuring leading horror actor Bela Lugosi. The film was a flop, but was later immortalized in a Tim Burton-directed biopic about the infamous director, played by Johnny Depp and which featured actress Lisa Marie as Nurmi.

Against the straitjacket of cultural conformity, and during a time when outward displays of female sexuality were discouraged, Nurmi's reinvention as a hellish temptress broke boundaries. Which is why, despite her star fading by the 60s, her impact on culture remains everlasting.

Chapter XII:
The goths and goth-coded: in their words, part III

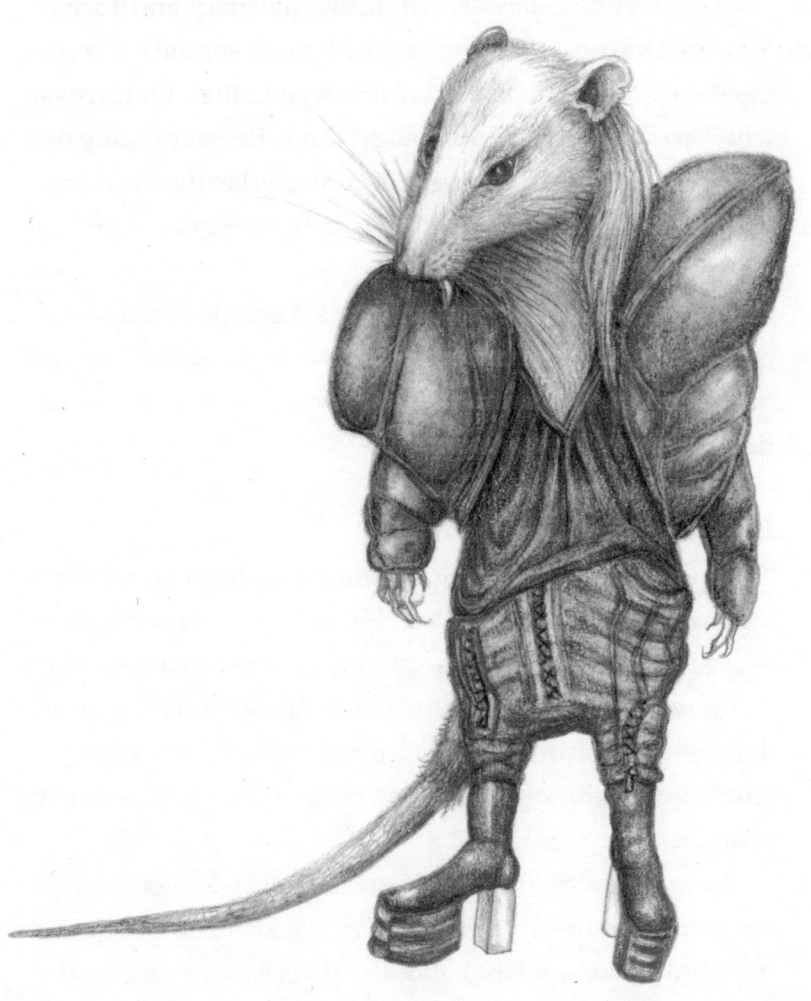

Kristina Nagel, artist

'For me, goth is a vibe and a mindset. Enjoying the morbid side of life and finding beauty in things others consider dark. Goth is not a phase. It is something that you either are or aren't. You don't have to wear black all the time. It doesn't make you a goth only by wearing black. I think you can perfectly wear white and identify as goth too. At least I do partly. I also do think culture is so fragmented these days, that you don't have to identify as goth fully anyway. It can be one or two aspects of your personality.

'When it comes to beauty choices, I stopped using black eyeliner since I got glasses but I never wear makeup or concealer to cover my dark eye circles, so I look most of the time a bit pale and unwell.'

Lynn Yaeger, fashion critic

'Goth to me is a very young person with a fierce uncompromising attitude. Lots of black, lots of rips and tears, lots of heavy makeup – but underneath you can sense a vulnerability and a sweetness. I think goth brings to fashion a very welcome darkness, a welcome respite from the very false sunniness and forced sexiness that fashion conglomerates believe will result in sales.

'I would describe my style as sort of cracked deconstructed doll/superannuated ballerina. I favour very big dresses with a tulle tutu hanging out the bottom – a shapeless smock is always my friend! It's something that I know is very distinctive, and it has been my style for decades.'

Martina Tiefenthaler, creative director
Goth [*noun*]
UK /ɡɒθ/
US /ˈɡɑː.θ/

'I was a teen in the late 90s and belonged to the hip hop and RnB scene. I dressed tight and oversized, sparkly, colourful and black. I had a very style-defining older brother and followed his lead. To me, goth was crazy and off, but I did not know it and judged by aesthetics only.

'Later in life I allowed my curiosity to unfold and experimented with various styles. Organically I ended up dressing almost exclusively in black, which might be the result of working with colours for so many years. Black is my uniform, it allows me to focus on creating a silhouette, and on curating a combination of textures, without any colour distraction. Black is neutral. I am somewhat of a shadow, a moving form.

'Darkness has always been part of fashion, throughout costume history; it had different meanings, though. It stood for purity and loyalty, as much as it stood for trust, elegance and competence. In the 16th century, dressing black was the most modern thing to do. Imagine the minimalism of the 90s without black. Now 30 years later people think I am goth, just because I dress dark and am naturally pale? I do not know much about the goth lifestyle actually, and I do not listen to its music, which is why I do not like to get called goth, I feel misunderstood and as if I am appropriating something that is not mine.

'Black dressing has a bad connotation in the mainstream today, unfortunately. Those who tell me I am goth seem to get sad about my looks, it drags them down. They think colour means joy and black means sadness. To me black means my absolute beautiful freedom.'

Michèle Lamy, artist, designer and muse

'There is a great beauty to darkness . . . mystery . . . magic. Goth is . . . punk, eclectic, junkie, skinny, excess, youth. Style is individuality. What you need is an attitude of always taking on challenges without being bound by preconceptions. Beauty is to belong. A way to express ourselves. For me, beauty is a journey. Things can come and go, but it is all going in the same direction, so I am very persistent in my pursuit of beauty.'

Pam Hogg, designer

'Even as a child, I was never drawn to "pretty things". I cross the two thresholds by combining sweet saccharine with darker elements. You'll never find me in a pair of nice shoes as I don't own any, I'm more of a masculine dresser, boots, braces and shirts kind of gal, with an occasional strapped shiny black high stiletto and dark stockings.'

Princess Julia, DJ

'My "gothicness" partly stems from being dumped in front of a black-and-white TV before colour screens had even entered our homes, where an education in imagery must have subliminally informed my consciousness. The allure of shadowy black-and-white film has always fascinated me. In my late teens, as part of the New Romantic movement, I attempted my own contoured look that took reference from early film noir and Surrealist art movements of the 20s onwards. I was obsessed, I was seeking a perfection of sorts. Creating a heavily made-up face that would photograph almost mask-like. Painfully shy, I used makeup to hide behind. Mid-70s punk was all about anti-fashion and confrontation, the New Romantics of the late 70s sought a kind of idealized perfection, which ultimately was also confrontational, but with a twist. There were elements of punk that blurred into our futuristic looks; it wasn't until the early 80s that "goth" truly became a thing, merging glam rock, punk and New Romantic elements.

'I think the allure of theatricality and a sense of occasion appealed to my feelings of otherness. I didn't feel I fitted into the life traditional society had in store for me. Gothic can be a look, but it's also a sensibility. It can be a wistful mood, melancholic, or relay a sense of decadence. It's a dark and mesmerizing aura, whether you're dressed up or dressed down. It's something to do with the doom and glamour of the human condition.'

Simone Rocha, designer

'I think the visceral feeling of darkness runs through us all and it's about harnessing that and expressing it in a way that feels powerful and provocative.

'For me, goth is the Central Bank in Temple Bar in Dublin where I used to hang out as a teenager.'

Susie Cave, designer

'I like goths. I always have. I like their quietness and I like their resilience – the fact that 40 years on from their beginnings, as a kind of Eeyorish aberration of the post-Punk movement, they still continue to walk the earth.

'What I love about gothic-ness in fashion is the explicit acknowledgement of the sadness of things. The darkness of the gothic look is often more expressive than words themselves; our exterior costume becomes the unspoken, yet eloquent expression of our hearts.

'My own creations in The Vampire's Wife, even though often floral or very colourful, still hold in their essence a sort of ethereal melancholy, they feel ghost-like, little levitations. They are dresses that concede the sorrow at the heart of the world, while rising defiantly above it. This for me is the spirit of gothic-ness. It is not depressive, it is not wallowing in darkness, rather it is a mutinous acknowledgement of the melancholy nature of things as a form of positive expression. I rarely wear black, but in my heart, there will always be a kind of defiant gothic-ness. My husband says that when the apocalypse finally comes all that will remain are the Goths! Long may they reign!'

Tali Lennox, artist

'The gothic elements I am most drawn to are from the past. I'm endlessly fascinated by history and imagining how people lived in centuries long gone. Living within a gothic aesthetic allows one to summon wonderment within the mystical and unknown. The objects or clothing we gather in our everyday can be a conduit to connecting to this romance of magic and *memento mori*: 19th-century black lace and corseted clothing, sourced black and white photographs, walks through the gothic tombs of Parisian cemeteries, my cave-like painting studio with intentionally minimal natural light, the church my boyfriend lives in, in England, or the old gothic town I resided in, in upstate New York, wildly designed old mansions, creaking floorboards, copula and fireplaces. I've certainly been told I have a "morbid curiosity", but I'm truly in love with the thrill of extracting the past from everyday moments.'

Chapter XIII:
Get in loser, we're going shopping

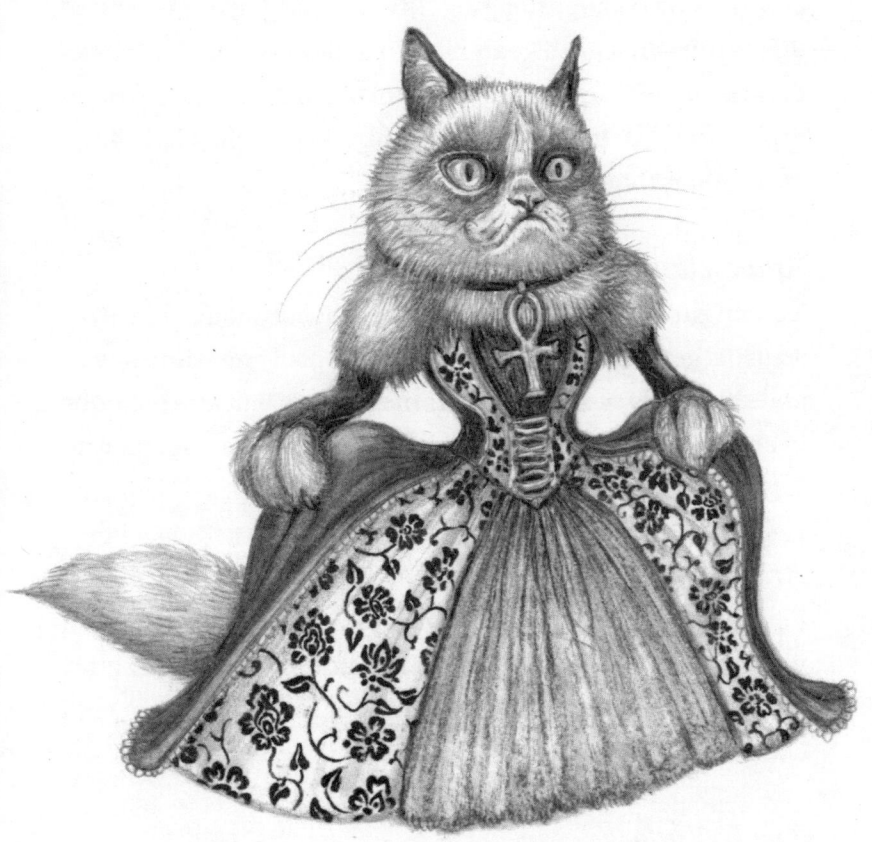

Part of the joy of putting together a wardrobe comes from cultivating a little black book of independent boutiques that you can call upon when you need a quick refresh. From vintage dealers touting Victorian mourning capes to obscure curio shops flogging futuristic athleisure wear and 90s minimalist goth gear, here to make your capitalist wet dreams come true is a list of some of the finest treasure troves to plunder while trying to navigate this so-called life. Get in loser, we're going shopping.

Annie's Ibiza
You might not think of this as the most obvious choice for aspiring goths, but once you get past the party girl rhinestones and shimmery sequin discs, Annie's Ibiza's Balearic boutique is crammed with Edwardian lace, antique capelets and Egyptian Revival Assuit.

Aralda
Founded by former model Brynn Jones, Aralda is LA's cult vintage boutique specializing in iconic 90s and noughties pieces, like McQueen's monochromatic houndstooth or John Galliano velvet devoré.

Atsuko Kudo
Atsuko Kudo is a London-based latex house where you can source anything from liquid-rubber trench coats to second-skin dresses with printed lace detailing. Buy custom-made or fresh off the racks, because every goth needs a latex moment.

Byronesque

Boasting hoards of obscure pieces, such as a leather capelet from Alexander McQueen's autumn/winter 1998 Joan of Arc collection, or 90s-era 'Lumps and Bumps' Commes, Byronesque's online shop curates some of the finest relics in fashion history.

Dead Lotus Couture

When it comes to latex, most brands lean into the integrity of the material as a kind of second skin, which is why the clothes are always cinched-in and body-con. Dead Lotus Couture does the exact opposite, using high shine, rubbery textures in the most unlikely shapes and uncanny silhouettes. Cue: oversized T-shirts, loose grandad cardigans and military-style cargo pants. Weirdly, these are even more perverse than their collection of bondage corsets and alien-esque body suits.

Eveliina Vintage

Run by LA-based dealers Eeva Musacchia and her twin daughters, Eveliina Vintage is a silky haven filled with cotton-candy negligées, peachy peignoirs and gorgeous organza gowns, making it a must-visit Mecca for any aspiring Lolita goth. That said, there are also plenty of black magic moments for those allergic to colour.

Falbalas

Named after Jacques Becker's fraught French film about a wayward fashion designer, Françoise and Erwan de Fligué's

Falbalas boutique is one of Paris's most prized possessions. Located in the Marché Dauphine, its walls are lined with exquisite antique corsetry and lace-up leather boots.

House of Harlot

From spiked rubber dresses to high-shine lingerie, add a fetishistic flourish to your armoury with beautifully crafted House of Harlot latex.

Illisa's Vintage Lingerie

Tucked away in the basement of Manhattan's Art and Antiques Center, Illisa's Vintage Lingerie is a slinky emporium filled with peppermint cream tap pants, lavender chiffon slips and champagne negligées. Perfect for your pastoral goth summer moments or layering under leather, it's where gothic goddess Tali Lennox gets all her silky numbers.

Jane Bourvis

From Irish crochet gowns with big bell sleeves to Normandy lace numbers with huge trains, Jane Bourvis's collection of antique wedding dresses lend a ghostly quality to any gothic bride-to-be. Nuptials aside, these dresses also make great partywear. Find her tucked away under the Westway in London's Portobello Green.

JHROP

From distressed Margiela Tabi boots to deconstructed Yohji Yamamoto tailoring, Hong Kong-based vintage boutique JHROP (pronounced 'drop') offers an expertly curated smorgasbord of 90s and noughties fashion for any goth looking to refine her look.

Matieres Fecales

Hell-raising art, fashion and music duo Fecal Matter are all about scaring the mainstream. They do this most successfully through their brand Matieres Fecales, which encompasses everything from straitjacket-inspired trench coats to oversized tees emblazoned with their demonic image.

Mowalola

Mixing the iconography of traditional horror – ghosts, bullet holes, crucifixes and bats – with notes of bondage and the tropes of the street, Nigerian designer Mowalola Ogunlesi makes hardcore clothes for hardcore people. Think oversized denim chaps, hoodies with built-in gimp masks and itsy-bitsy leather briefs.

Nymfa

There's a certain fustiness that comes with vintage clothing, but not when it's as expertly curated as it is at Nymfa's Brussels-based boutique. Sourced by former designer Ondine Patout, 90s-era multi-zipper Miu Miu skirts and paired-back Ann Demeulemeester separates take on a distinctly modern feel.

OOTO Archive

With showrooms across London, Los Angeles and Dallas, Out Of The Ordinary Archive is your go-to destination for

Tom Ford-era Gucci. Not just the shop floor stuff either, I'm talking real runway pieces like his show-stopping jersey gowns with their strategically placed cut-outs and peekaboo metalwork or his bondage-inspired twin sets with bra strap detailing.

Online Ceramics

Online Ceramics is the cult online clothing brand from Alix Ross and Elijah Funk. Creating spooky streetwear for ghoul girls and horror movie buffs, over the past few years they've teamed up with a motley crew of collaborators including Heaven by Marc Jacobs, dark temptress Dilara Findikoglu, A24 (the production company behind chilling flicks *Midsommar* (2019), *Hereditary* (2018) and *The Witch* (2015)) and New Age spiritualist Ram Dass.

Opulent Addict

From steampunky Jean Paul Gaultier to 90s-era Dolce bondage, Opulent Addict is the go-to destination for that specifically stygian brand of glamour.

Pretty Box Boutique

Visiting Paris's Pretty Box Boutique is like falling down the rabbit hole and waking up at a BDSM rave meets UFO convention. The walls are lined with military gas masks, rubber aliens and some of the finest vintage Paris has to offer, from rare Junya Watanabe and 30s cobweb lace to gothabilly band The Cramps memorabilia and latex sailor jackets from unknown designers.

PRODUCTS.LTD

With her latest creative offering Products.Ltd, creative director Betsy Johnson gives streetwear a brooding, futuristic twist. Think nylon leggings worn with matching muffs, belts emblazoned with the word 'sale' and big-skirted fishtail gowns made from patchworked football shirts.

Rebecca Sweeting

From 19th-century bonnets and velvet chokers adorned with antique buckles to Victorian mourning mantels with intricate jet beading, Rebecca Sweeting's East London studio is an Aladdin's cave of relics from the past. You can also find her every Friday at Portobello Green Market.

Second Skin Archive

Avant-garde with an element of distress, but also crisp and clean in the way she puts it all together, Millie Foster Price's online shop Second Skin Archive is as much a reflection of her personal style and taste as it is a celebration of vintage fashion. From lesser-known Japanese designers like Nozomi Ishiguro to the rarest of 90s-era Vivienne Westwood, you can find almost anything in her extraordinary archive.

Strogo

Sourcing everything from 20s embellished slips to no-label 90s leather, Russian-based boutique Strogo Vintage is your one-stop destination for all things vintage. Ideal for lazy goths who don't like shopping around.

The Corner Store

Founded by designer, stylist and gothic siren Stacey Nishimoto, The Corner Store is a digital treasure trove of dark and romantic one-off pieces like embroidered tulle veils by Geoffrey Beene or charcoal Blumarine slips.

Timeless Vixen

Founded by otherworldly vamp Lauren Lepire, Timeless Vixen is the LA-based treasure trove specializing in one-of-a-kind pieces, whether that's a figure-hugging Alaïa number fit for a modern-day Morticia or a slinky Galliano bias-cut dress.

Turner Vintage

Shani Turner has been collecting vintage pieces since she was a teenager. An expert in Egyptian Revival Assuit and gossamer-fine lace from the 30s, her Portobello Market stall is one of London's best-kept secrets (until now). Ideal for adding a bit of faded grandeur to your wardrobe.

Chapter XIV:
How to live like a goth

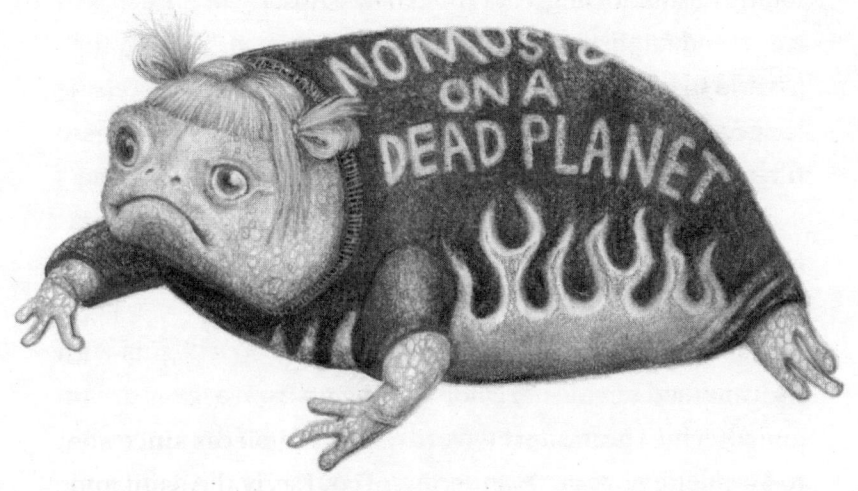

Honing your style is only part of the story. The rest comes from the world you build around you: the films you watch, the music you listen to, the books you read and the physical space you inhabit. Because being goth isn't just about how you look, it's a way of life – which means it's time to get holistic. To totally misquote the great 19th-century American thinker and transcendentalist leader Ralph Waldo Emerson: 'To be goth in a world that is constantly trying to make you something else is the greatest accomplishment'. So here are some suggestions to fill in the rest of the blanks.

HOW TO DO UP A HOUSE, HAUNTED OR OTHERWISE

Daphne du Maurier's 1938 gothic novel *Rebecca* begins with its unnamed female narrator waking up from a fever dream and uttering the immortal words: 'Last night I dreamt I went to Manderley again.' Manderley, of course, is the handsome estate she has become chatelaine to after shacking up with the mysterious widower Maxim de Winter. Despite its beauty, the house has become a shrine to Rebecca, the first Mrs de Winter, who supposedly died in a boating accident and whose memory is kept alive by Mrs Danvers, the creepy housekeeper who is devoted to her former mistress. Much of the book's action occurs within these haunted walls, making Manderley a central narrative device, which is very typical of the genre.

Indeed, within the canon of gothic literature, houses were more than just foreboding backdrops: they took on anthropomorphic tendencies, becoming sinister characters in their own right. There's the crumbling pad in Edgar Allan Poe's *The Fall of the House of Usher* (1839), whose fate is tied to its equally decrepit inhabitants. There's also Miss Havisham's decaying digs in *Great Expectations* (1861), Wuthering Heights in Emily Brontë's *Wuthering Heights* (1847), Bluebeard's not-so-humble abode in Angela Carter's *The Bloody Chamber* (1979), and Manfred's gothic seat in Horace Walpole's *The Castle of Otranto* (1764), with its secret passageways and hidden trapdoors. In fact, such was his gothic kink, that Walpole spent over 30 years finessing the art of 'gloomth', a word he coined to describe the atmosphere at Strawberry Hill, the gothic revival fort he built just outside London, replete with pinnacles, stained glass windows, battlements, vaulted ceilings and a round tower.

We can't all live in a rotting gothic castle. After all, we gothic creatures like our creature comforts. But that doesn't mean we can't gothify the place that we call home. No matter where you live – Victorian townhouse, mid-century villa, pied-à-terre, bachelorette pad, belfry, mud hut, hovel – how you do up your physical surroundings is a direct representation of who you are. It reflects your tastes, sensibilities and even your aspirations. Someone who understood that assignment was Luisa Casati, who used to decorate every hotel room she ever stayed in with a menagerie of animal skins, exotic plumes, mechanical songbirds and magic trinkets. It's a similar story for singer Ethel Cain, who has lived in a different house every year since leaving home. Whether it's an abandoned 19th-century church in rural Indiana or a wood-panelled mid-century dwelling in Alabama, each place is rendered in her signature Southern gothic style, replete with deer skulls, china dolls, framed dead insects, crucifixes and a vintage star-spangled banner, a symbol of America's dark underbelly.

There was a moment in 2020 when every interior trending on Instagram seemed to merge into one, a hall of mirrors characterized by millennial pink walls, indoor plants in hanging baskets, cloud-like modular sofas in black leather or white bouclé, and a tyranny of tutti-frutti terrazzo, inspired by the old Celine shops. If your dwelling didn't look like the backdrop of a Glossier campaign or a bar of nougat, what business did you have even living there? Of course, each to their own. But tapping into the tropes of Good Taste simply because you're unsure of how else to do it, or because that's how everyone else is doing it, feels at odds with the bigger picture you're trying to project, which is one of fearlessness, individualism and irreverence, coupled with a healthy dose of darkness and eccentricity.

When it came to doing up my own space, I wanted there to be some kind of tension. I'm a sucker for faded grandeur, but always tempered by something modern: A mid-century Japanese washi paper lamp juxtaposed with an antique verdure tapestry I haggled over at Kempton Market. A 50s chain sconce hung above a 19th-century plaster bust or a piece of medieval armour I found in some village shop. For me, it's about having an eclectic mix of curiosities, the kind that you might find at a yard sale for a haunted house (although the only things I'm haunted by are the lots I miss out on at auction).

Of course, you can still be a maximalist without opting for antiques. For example, Erykah Badu transformed her Dallas studio home into a witchy shrine filled with Buddhas, tuning forks and African masks. Similarly, you can embrace antiques without going full maximalist. Amanda Harlech recently restored Glyn Cywarch, a 17th-century Jacobean manor in north Wales, to its former bare-boned glory. Salvaged wooden panelling and humongous smoky oak fireplaces run throughout the house, while the chalky white walls are punctuated with the odd ancestral portrait or heraldic crest. Or you can do something else entirely. For example, Michèle Lamy's Paris apartment – the former headquarters of the French Socialist Party – is a lesson in raw brutalist beauty, with its vast concrete features, horned furniture and monstrous raised platform bed, which she makes as part of OWENSCORP.

The point here is that there are myriad ways to do up your place, as long as it's a true representation of who you are. Which means the best advice is to simply identify your quirk, lean into it and have fun.

INTERIORS CHECKLIST: THE ESSENTIALS

Taxidermy

The physical impossibility of death in the mind of someone living. It doesn't get much more morbid than adorning your home with dead animals, a practice that was first introduced in ancient Egyptian times, although this was less of a *World of Interiors* flex and more to do with preserving the memory of beloved pets and bringing them with you into the afterlife. Meanwhile, using exotic hides as a form of bedding was popular among early European and Native American societies. It wasn't until the Renaissance era, however, that taxidermy was first embraced as an art form, and collecting animal skins and skeletons became a cultural pursuit.

It goes without saying: any animal matter you use to decorate your home today needs to be antique. No animals were harmed during the making of this gothic abode. Furthermore, if the thought of transforming your home into a pet cemetery feels too Stephen King, there are ways of tapping into the trend without going the whole hog. For example, you can opt for a wall of framed butterflies like the architect and photographer Carlo Mollino, whose hidden Turin home should already be on your Pinterest moodboard. An even subtler option would be to garnish a credenza with a vase of exotic plumes, an ornamental ostrich egg or a majestic moose antler as a nod to Michèle Lamy. And if you really can't stomach it, you can always do it the vegan way with a smattering of animal prints.

Shrines and religious ephemera

Ingrained within the gothic tradition is the appropriation/subversion of religious iconography, whether that means wearing a crucifix around your neck or decorating your ears with ankhs. The same applies to the home. For example, furnishing the walls with great big crosses or fashioning small shrines replete with Buddhas, sound bowls and sage. In fact, there's nothing witchier than having your own domestic altar – something you can do with antique fonts, ex-votos, reliquaries and altarpieces – the more obscure and folky the better. You can also throw in some wavy, spiral or zig-zag metal candlesticks (see interior designer Jermaine Gallacher) and an assortment of crystals and spiced incense to double down on the crypt-like atmosphere. And even some *memento mori*, such as an ornamental skull or some dried flowers. Think of this space as a sanctuary where you can go to put a hex on an ex-lover or bad boss, manifest your dream job or contemplate the fragility of the human condition. You know, the quotidian stuff.

Ancestral portraits

What would Dorian Gray be without his portrait? Probably much better off, but then there would be no story. Faustian pact aside, adorning the home with an ancestral (yours, or anyone else's for that matter) portrait is a key characteristic of the gothic home. It's a great way to add a sense of history and theatre and to take up some of that wall space. Just think of the ghosts attached to them.

Shells

Among the many other gothic tropes that make up Strawberry Hill, one of Horace Walpole's favourite features was a garden bench or love seat which he had made in the shape of a shell. Because, when it comes to *objets d'art*, there's no better artist than Mother Nature. Indeed, shells, coral and other natural forms are a great way to furnish a home. Tuck a giant clam shell under a console or embellish a window sill with a sprawling sea fan, or get creative and fix a smattering of mottled scallop shells to a skirting board or mirror frame. It's all about channelling the sublime beauty of nature, which at its heart is incredibly gothic: think grotto drama meets sea-witch chic. It's also highly affordable: simply buy a bag of shells on Etsy or head to your nearest beach with a vampiric tote.

Tapestries

Whether it's a wall pieced together with verdure fragments or a great big hunt scene suspended from the ceiling, tapestries create an immediate sense of faded grandeur. So enamoured by them were the late Isabella Blow and her husband that they had entire walls devoted to them at their Arts and Crafts home Hilles House. Age-worn (the more distressed the better), their rich patina will either chime in with the rest of your antiques or jar beautifully with something industrial and modern like exposed concrete or metal work. Add another layer by hanging a mirror or artwork on top of it.

Armour

There's nothing like a piece of armour or antique weaponry to set a sinister tone for wherever it is you're living. Like the film version of his brooding and chivalrous creation, Gomez Addams, cartoonist Charles Addams used to hang medieval crossbows on the walls of his two-storey Midtown penthouse in Manhattan, which was also home to a Civil War-era embalming table that he had fashioned into a coffee table. Talk about macabre.

Dark and romantic, these relics from a bygone era add a timeless quality to any space, whether that's a pair of shield sconces or an ornamental piece of chainmail. And if you're more of a pacifist, a simple piece of heraldry will provide the same effect.

WHAT TO WATCH: GOTHS ON FILM

Intrinsic to figuring out who you are is seeing yourself reflected back at you, and cinema plays an essential role in this. Think of it as your Lacanian *stade du miroir* (mirror moment); a form of mastery over the self. For me, this came courtesy of watching *The Addams Family* (1991) at the formative age of 11. Being welcomed into a family who delight in all things scary and spooky was like being seen for the first time. As a goth, there's no better way to come to terms with your shadow self than by watching those who revel in theirs – no greater feeling than what comes with discovering a film that resonates with those creeping feelings of sadness or otherness. So, from tales about teen hellraisers to parables about ageing misanthropes, below is a list of some of the best goth films to soothe your aching anxieties.

A Fool There Was (1915)

One of the very few surviving films starring cinema's original femme fatale Theda Bara, *A Fool There Was* is an American silent movie about a Wall Street hotshot and all-round family man who abandons his family and social standing after falling under the spell of a psychic vampire he meets on a ship, who uses her powers over men to subject them to ruin.

The Cabinet of Dr. Caligari (1920)

Coming out of the German Expressionist movement, *The Cabinet of Dr. Caligari* is a surreal silent movie about a mysterious doctor and his strange somnambulist sidekick, around whom murderous events start to unfurl. With its surreal set and innovative use of special effects, it is widely considered the first great work of the horror genre.

Un Chien Andalou (1929)

Directed by Spanish filmmaker Luis Buñuel, co-written by artist Salvador Dalí, and inspired by Freud's theories of free association and the subconscious, *Un Chien Andalou* is a scintillating masterpiece of Surrealist cinema. The silent movie opens with a disjointed dream-like sequence, featuring an image of the moon being bisected by a thin cloud, which is violently interspersed with a scene of a woman being held by a man, a razor hovering over her eye. With no real plot line, the film jumps frantically from one disturbing vignette to the next. Not the best idea to watch if you're already feeling a bit anxious.

The House on Haunted Hill (1959)

A classic haunted house B movie, *The House on Haunted Hill* stars Vincent 'King of Horror' Price as the eccentric millionaire Frederick Loren who invites a group of five strangers to spend the night in a spooky mansion in return for a cash prize. As it quickly becomes apparent, the house party is not alone.

Suddenly, Last Summer (1959)

Based on Tennessee Williams's Southern Gothic play, *Suddenly, Last Summer* is about a delirious young woman (Elizabeth Taylor) who has been institutionalized after witnessing the brutal death of her cousin Sebastian the previous summer, and her wealthy socialite aunt (Katharine Hepburn) who will stop at nothing to prevent those mysterious events coming to light. Note the excellent use of hats.

Whatever Happened to Baby Jane? (1962)

Starring doyennes of the silver screen Bette Davis and Joan Crawford, *Whatever Happened to Baby Jane?* is a psychological thriller about two rival sisters and fading Hollywood actresses Jane (Davis) and Blanche (Crawford) who spend their days tormenting each other in their decaying Hollywood mansion. Resentful of having to take care of the more famous, but wheelchair-bound Blanche, and desperate to revive her once illustrious career, Jane comes up with a dastardly plan.

Onibaba (1964)

Set during the Onin War in medieval Japan, *Onibaba* follows the story of a cunning old woman (Nobuko Otowa) and her young daughter-in-law (Jitsuko Yoshimura) who survive their bleak reality by murdering samurai soldiers and looting their dead bodies, trading their bounty with the town's local merchant. One day they meet a man in a demonic mask who they subsequently murder, and the old woman takes the mask for herself, only to find that the mask has a mind of its own.

Rosemary's Baby (1969)

Roman Polanski's psychological horror film brings to life what every mother has nightmares about: giving birth to the devil. Set in New York, newlyweds Guy (John Cassavetes) and Rosemary Woodhouse (Mia Farrow) have just moved into an apartment building when they are befriended by their mysterious elderly neighbours who have big, satanic plans for the young couple.

The Wicker Man (1973)

Sergeant Neil Howie (Edward Woodward) arrives on a remote Scottish island to investigate the disappearance of a young girl. While there, he becomes horrified by the strange pagan rituals practised by the villagers, which include shagging in bushes, sinister masked processions and suspected human sacrifice. Great inspiration for summer dressing.

Picnic at Hanging Rock (1975)

Picnic at Hanging Rock is a strange tale about a group of school girls at a strict Australian boarding school who are let out one afternoon for a Valentine's Day picnic at a prehistoric geological formation called Hanging Rock. After inextricably falling into a deep sleep, three girls and one teacher are reawakened and begin to climb the crevice in a trance-like state, until they vanish completely.

Carrie (1976)

A classic tale of misunderstood femininity, we are all Carrie at some point in our lives. Played by Sissy Spacek, Carrie White is a shy 16-year-old with telekinetic powers who lives with her fanatically religious mother. Bullied by her classmates, she is eventually invited to prom where she becomes the victim of a cruel prank, involving copious amounts of pig blood. The traumatic event triggers a psychotic breakdown, causing Carrie to use her powers as she seeks out her revenge.

The Hunger (1983)

The Hunger tells the horny tale of a human–vampire love triangle, featuring Miriam Blaylock (Catherine Deneuve) a YSL-wearing temptress who feasts upon the blood of the young by slashing their necks with a bladed ankh pendant, her hunky vampire lover John (David Bowie), whose rapidly ageing body is causing him some concern, and Sarah Roberts, (Susan Sarandon), the butch doctor of sleep disorders and unsuspecting object of Miriam's desire.

The Lost Boys (1987)

Possibly one of the best vampire movies ever made, *The Lost Boys* follows a pair of brothers, Michael (Jason Patric) and Sam (Corey Haim), as they move to Santa Carla, a small beach town overrun by a gang of teenage vampires who drive around on bikes and look exceptionally good in leather. In a bid to fit in with the cool gang and impress their leader David (Kiefer

Sutherland), Michael undergoes a series of initiations, with bloodthirsty consequences.

Beetlejuice (1988)

Recently deceased couple Barbara (Geena Davis) and Adam Maitland (Alec Baldwin) find their lives – or rather deaths – turned upside down when the painfully obnoxious Deetzes and their morose teen daughter Lydia (Winona Ryder) move into their house. Unable to scare them away, they call upon the services of a menacing spirit named Beetlejuice (Michael Keaton).

The Heathers (1988)

The Heathers is a black comedy about a monocle-wearing misanthrope named Veronica Sawyer (Winona Ryder) who becomes part of a popular girl gang where everybody is named Heather. Sick of the gang's bullying antics, she befriends the cool and sexy J D (Christian Slater), and together they start teaching the Heathers a dark lesson.

Bram Stoker's Dracula (1992)

Starring Gary Oldman as Count Dracula, the film follows the famed nightwalker as he journeys to England in search of Mina Harker (Winona Ryder), who he believes is the reincarnation of his long-lost lover Elizabeth. With spectacular costumes created by renowned costume designer Eiko Ishioka (from the voluminous lace headdress and collar inspired by the ruffles of a lizard's neck worn by Sadie Frost, to the diaphanous drapery worn by Dracula's brides), Francis Ford Coppola's highly camp but beautifully macabre masterpiece is what goth dreams are made of.

The Crow (1994)

Based on the comic book series of the same name, *The Crow* is a brooding revenge story starring the late Brandon Lee as Eric Draven, a rock musician killed in an attack that also saw the brutal rape and murder of his fiancée Shelly (Sofia Shinas). Resurrected by a mysterious crow, with whom he shares telepathic powers, Eric sets out to avenge their deaths. Another love letter to men wearing leather.

The Doom Generation (1995)

Two horny, tripped-out teens, Jordan White (James Duval) and Amy Blue (Rose McGowan), pick up a hunky drifter named Xavier Red (Johnathon Schaech) one night while driving home from a club in Gregg Araki's lurid coming-of-age tale. After a fight at a corner store turns deadly, the three find themselves on the run around LA's cesspits, and experience various violent encounters along the way.

The Craft (1996)

An important coming-of-age film for any nascent goth, *The Craft* follows Sarah Bailey (Robin Tunney), a teen misfit with telekinetic powers and new kid on the block, who joins a coven of wannabe witches, and together they start to wreak havoc on their school. Things take a turn when Nancy (Fairuza Balk), the group's leader, is unable to quench her thirst for power. Watch this for style tips alone.

Thirst (2009)

Loosely based on the 1867 novel *Thérèse Raquin* by Émile Zola, *Thirst* is a desperate story about a lonely Catholic priest suffering from feelings of self-doubt, who becomes the unwitting victim of a scientific experiment gone wrong while trying to find a cure for a deadly virus. After being injected with the virus and given a blood transfusion, Sang-hyun (Song Kang-ho) makes a miraculous recovery, causing villagers to flock to him to seek out his supposedly magical healing powers. The only problem is that Sang-hyun has suddenly developed a taste for human blood.

Jennifer's Body (2009)

Jennifer's Body is about an unlikely friendship between Jennifer Check (Megan Fox), the hottest girl in school, and Anita Lesnicki (Amanda Seyfried), her nerdy sidekick. One night, after going to see their favourite band play, Jennifer gets abducted by the band and sacrificed as a virgin in return for fame and fortune. Because these days making it as an indie band requires a blood sacrifice. The only problem is that Jennifer isn't a virgin. Instead, she turns into a sexy succubus, develops superhuman powers and starts feeding on male human flesh, much to Anita's chagrin.

The Witch (2015)

Set in the 17th century, a Puritan settler family arrives at the edge of a forest to begin their new life. One day, while

Thomasin (Anya Taylor-Joy) is playing with her baby brother in the woods, he suddenly and inexplicably vanishes. More children go missing and the family becomes aware of the presence of a witch.

Get Out (2017)

Jordan Peele's psychological horror film will chill you to your bones. Chris Washington (Daniel Kaluuya) is a young photographer who travels to upstate New York to stay with his girlfriend Rose's (Allison Williams) family. Though everything appears normal at first, Chris becomes increasingly disturbed by the comments Rose's family and their friends continue to make about Black people. Even more disturbing is the strange, vacant behaviour of the few Black people within the community. It doesn't take long for Chris to realize he needs to get the fuck out of there.

Suspiria (2018)

It's rare when a remake is as good as the original, but that is most definitely the case with Luca Guadagnino's reinterpretation of Dario Argento's 1977 cult classic. The bone-curdling events of *Suspiria* take place at the Markos Dance Academy in West Berlin, where American student Susie Bannion (Dakota Johnson) has just been enrolled. When she arrives, the school is still dealing with the disappearance of a young dancer, who before she went missing confided in her therapist that the academy was being run by a coven of witches, most of whom are played by Tilda Swinton in various forms of disguise. A struggle for witchy supremacy ensues.

Midsommar (2019)

Ari Aster's chilling film is as much about a breakup as it is about a bloodthirsty pagan cult. The plot follows a bunch of American students as they journey to Scandinavia to visit the Hårga festival. Dani (Florence Pugh) and Christian (Jack Reynor) have been drifting apart for a few months now, while Dani is still reeling from the trauma of her family's murder-suicide at the hands of her bipolar sister. Unbeknownst to them, however, the crux of the festival revolves around a sling of ritualistic human sacrifices and the nomination of a May Queen to preside over it all.

Pearl (2022)

Co-written by Ti West and actress Mia Goth, *Pearl* is the second instalment of West's slasher trilogy, and the backstory to the events that take place in *X* (2022). Set on a rural Texan farm during the 1918 influenza pandemic, *Pearl* follows a young woman (Goth) desperate for fame, resentful of her husband, who is away fighting in World War I, and suffering from burgeoning psychopathic tendencies.

WHAT TO LISTEN TO: A VERY GOTHIC PLAYLIST

Entombed within the gothic condition are feelings of pain and anguish – no matter your age or your circumstance. Thankfully, however, musicians have been channelling these emotions into powerful ballads, maudlin musings, fevered requiems and thrashing metal synths for centuries. A lot of the songs below have nothing to do with goth in the traditional sense; some came before the genre's inception, while others came after. But they are all connected by a shared emotional experience, the experience of feeling, in some way, dark or 'other'. So put a record on and, in the words of Andrew Eldritch, dance the ghost with me.

George Frideric Handel, 'Sarabande', 1703–6

Inspired by a controversial 16th-century dance from Central America that was banned in most countries for its obscenity, Handel's 'Sarabande' is the fourth movement of his Keyboard suite in D minor. Considered among the great works of the Baroque period, it slipped into obscurity until Stanley Kubrick revived it in his scintillating historical drama, *Barry Lyndon* (1975).

Wolfgang Amadeus Mozart, Don Giovanni 'Overture', 1784

The cautionary tale of Don Juan, the legendary libertine who meets his infernal fate, is brought to life via Mozart's thundering overture. It's also used to represent Mozart's scary dad in Miloš Forman's sumptuous classic *Amadeus* (1984).

Giuseppe Verdi, Requiem, 1874

Inspired by the Roman Catholic tradition of honouring the dead with Gregorian chants, Verdi's *Requiem* is a powerful masterpiece that beautifully articulates the grief and sorrow the composer felt after the death of Italian writer and nationalist Alessandro Manzoni.

Claude Debussy, The Fall of the House of Usher, *1908–17*

In *The Fall of the House of Usher,* French composer Claude Debussy's flesh-crawling strings breathe life into Edgar Allan Poe's dismal tale about a rotting mansion and its mysterious, moribund inhabitants.

Screamin' Jay Hawkins, 'I Put a Spell on You', 1956

'I Put a Spell on You' was meant to be a traditional blues ballad, but Screamin' Jay Hawkins got drunk at the recording studio and ended up grunting and moaning his way through the macabre song. The resulting track was deemed so outrageous that it was banned from most radio programming. Leaning into the song's diabolical nature, Hawkins would take to the stage in occulty nose tusks and a long cape, rising out of a coffin that was shrouded in smoke.

The Rolling Stones, 'Paint It Black', 1966

The Rolling Stones' 'Paint It Black' is about staring out at the world's vibrancy and only seeing black; a metaphor for the depression and numbness that comes with searing grief and sudden loss, it went on to influence generations of angsty artists from the goth movement and beyond.

The Velvet Underground, 'All Tomorrow's Parties', 1967

With its funereal sounds and nihilistic lyrics about a lost creature of the night shrouded in darkness and wearing a ragged, silky gown (words that could conjure any number of vampy vixens featured in this book), 'All Tomorrow's Parties', by pop culture's black-clad anti-heroes The Velvet Underground, perfectly encapsulates the grim realities of Warhol's New York.

The Doors, 'Riders on the Storm', 1971
Riddled with foreboding fragments about dogs without bones and actors out on loan, The Doors' proto-gothic 'Riders on the Storm' gives an accurate portrayal of post-60s America and a paranoia about its loss of innocence.

Bauhaus, 'Bela Lugosi's Dead', 1979
High priests of darkness, Bauhaus are largely credited with kicking off the entire undead movement. They did this most mesmerizingly with 'Bela Lugosi's Dead'. Named after 20s horror film star Bela Lugosi, it's a chilling nine-minute celebration of all things scary and spooky, against a backdrop of ominous guitar strings and Peter Murphy's disturbed vocals.

The Cure, 'A Forest', 1980
Evoking perturbed images of a dark abyss, as well as the idea of chasing something that isn't there, the urgent ramblings of Robert Smith paint an agonizing picture of a goth in distress.

Joy Division, 'Atmosphere', 1980
With its melancholic musings about abandonment and self-loathing, set to Ian Curtis's quasi-operatic warbling and Stephen Morris's sombre beats, Joy Division's maudlin anthem is a true reflection of the goth experience.

Soft Cell, 'Tainted Love', 1981

Juxtaposing jumpy synths with eerie vocals and angsty lyrics, Soft Cell's 'Tainted Love' tells the tale of a romance gone bad.

Siouxsie and the Banshees, 'Spellbound', 1981

The music video for Siouxsie and the Banshees' 'Spellbound' opens with an ominous vision of a prowling cat overlayed with an image of a leathered-up Sioux hypnotically crawling on all fours while a purple curtain burns in the background, before a woodland chase scene unfolds as the band flees from a masked witch. Fraught and frenzied, it is one of the greatest gothic anthems of the period.

Klaus Nomi, 'The Cold Song', 1983

German countertenor and surreal performance artist Klaus Nomi was celebrated as much for his impressive vocal range as he was for his macabre makeup and otherworldly stage theatrics. His eerily beautiful live performance of 'The Cold Song', taken from Henry Purcell and John Dryden's *King Arthur* opera, in which he sings the words 'I can scarcely move/ Or draw my breath . . . Let me, let me/Freeze again to death!' is made ever more poignant by the fact that he died a few months later as a result of an AIDS-related illness.

The Cramps, 'Human Fly', 1983

Gothabilly band The Cramps' psychedelic track 'Human Fly' tells the absurd tale of an anthropomorphized fly buzzing about the place, as a metaphor for the self-indulgent misfit.

The Sisters of Mercy, 'Lucretia My Reflection', 1985

In some ways, 'Lucretia My Reflection' is a love letter to sexy goth sirens throughout the ages, from Italian noblewoman Lucrezia Borgia, after whom the song is named, to new band member Patricia Morrison, to whom it is unofficially dedicated. But it's also a battle cry for the disenfranchized to rise up against oppressive governments and big corporations, amid a sonic landscape of throbbing beats and Andrew Eldritch's menacing vocals.

The Damned, 'Eloise', 1986

Blending elements of punk rock, pop and new wave with Dave Vanian's lugubrious vocals, The Damned's rendition of 'Eloise' is a mournful and melodramatic song about pining after some chick named Eloise. Despite being the band's biggest-ever chart success, they were never allowed to make a music video (possibly to do with stubborn record company bosses and shrinking budgets). Luckily, however, a recording exists of a live performance featuring a white-clad Vanian replete with romantic pirate shirt, high-waisted pants and sinister but sexy white gloves.

The Cranberries, 'Zombie', 1994

Despite being written about The Troubles in Northern Ireland, there's something incredibly universal about the fury with which Irish rock band The Cranberries use to describe the atrocities of the 1993 Warrington bombing. In her screeching repetition of the lyrics 'in your head', frontwoman Dolores O'Riordan's pain is raw and palpable.

Garbage, 'Milk', 1996

With lyrics like 'I am weak/But I am strong', Shirley Manson's hypnotic hymn about aching for a lost lover perfectly sums up the paradoxical feelings of heartbreak and longing.

Placebo, 'Every Me Every You', 1999

From agitated guitar strings to dark overlord Brian Molko's snarling, nasal vocals to lyrics about broken bodies and poison coming undone, Placebo's 'Every Me Every You' is the ultimate teen goth anthem. The fact that it plays at the beginning credits of cult film *Cruel Intentions* (1999) while the camera pans from an American graveyard to the brooding Sebastian driving along in his hearse of a Jaguar, is a testament to that.

The Horrors, 'Who Can Say', 2009

Heirs to the great gothic canon, The Horrors were to millennials what Bauhaus was to Boomers' Britain. Celebrated for their particularly spooky brand of indie sleaze, 'Who Can Say' combines frantic post-punk chords with introspective lyrics about the fragility of identity and the societal pressures to conform.

Yung Lean, 'Hennessy & Sailor Moon', 2016

Yung Lean makes music you want to cry to. With its dreamy soundscape and lyrics about being haunted by a lover whose feelings might not be genuine, 'Hennessy & Sailor Moon' is no different.

Bladee ft Ecco2K, 'Obedient', 2018

Hazy and ethereal, listening to Drain Gang members Bladee and Ecco2K rap about the pain of simply existing feels like falling through a cloud while high on Xanax.

FKA twigs, 'Cellophane', 2019

Blending breathy vocals with maudlin piano chords and heart-wrenching lyrics about not being good enough, FKA twigs's hauntingly beautiful 'Cellophane' is a brutal portrayal of a withering relationship.

Arca ft No Bra, 'Witch', 2021

Words can't accurately do justice to the mind-melting magic and surreal beauty of Arca's 'Witch'. A song about monsters, mortals, witches and machines, it's about the fluidity of identity and the tension between empowerment and subjugation.

Lana Del Rey, 'Season of the Witch', 2021

It was the filmmaker Guillermo del Toro's idea to have Lana Del Rey cover Donovan's 1966 classic 'Season of the Witch', which he then used for the soundtrack of his supernatural horror flick *Scary Stories to Tell in the Dark* (2019). With her velvety vocals coupled with Donovan's unsettling lyrics, the result was even more haunting than he'd imagined.

Ethel Cain, 'Family Tree', 2022

Merging *memento mori* symbols – nooses, crosses and bones – with weighty religious references, Ethel Cain's brooding

211

example of sludge metal captures the burning anguish of adolescence.

Yves Tumor, 'God is a Circle', 2022

'God is a Circle' is a nightmarish song about a toxic relationship spiralling out of control and into the depths of darkness.

Doja Cat, 'Demons', 2023

'Demons' is an uncanny blending of blistering beats, satanic lyrics and the rapper's signature sugary vocals. The accompanying music video, in which she appears as a hellish figure to torment scream queen Christina Ricci, is just as scary.

WHAT TO READ: GRIMOIRES TO FLICK THROUGH

In a world saturated with images, we often forget about the importance of the written word, with its ability to conjure people, places and things. Words are like spells, working within the parameters of your imagination to teleport you to another universe, which is why reading a book can be a totally transformative experience. In fact, there's no better feeling than poring over a piece of text and discovering something new, entirely for yourself, deep within the dark crevices of your mind, and knowing that no two readings are ever the same. And that's just books in general. Those with gothic inclinations are like that but on crack. Whether you're immersing yourself in the art of Crowley's black magic, or being confronted with images of decaying mansions or an orgy of severed eyeballs, books containing nefarious matter have the power to shock, confront and terrify you to your core, and sometimes even titillate you, making you question everything you think you know about yourself and the world you live in as a result. So without further ado, here is a list of grimoires to do exactly that. The library is now open.

Christopher Marlowe, Doctor Faustus, *1593*
The original Faustian pact: a young doctor makes a deal with the devil for knowledge and power over the demon Mephistopheles in return for his body and soul.

Horace Walpole, The Castle of Otranto, *1764*
The first ever gothic novel, *The Castle of Otranto* is a story about an ancient prophecy, ghostly apparitions and a man's desperate attempt to preserve his line.

Marquis de Sade, Juliette, *1797–1801*
A manifesto on sadism and depravity, de Sade's *Juliette* follows a young girl's moral decline and the pleasure she derives from it in the process.

Edgar Allan Poe, The Black Cat, *1843*
The Black Cat is a dark tale about a former feline lover turned cat (and wife!) murderer awaiting execution on death row. More than just RSPCA propaganda, it is a warning against the dangers of alcoholism.

Charles Baudelaire, Les Fleurs du Mal, *1857*

Baudelaire was into some seriously freaky stuff. An important work of the Symbolist movement, *Les Fleurs Du Mal* is a collection of morbid poetry about wooing vampires, sympathy for the devil and necrophiliac tendencies towards a putrifying corpse.

Charlotte Perkins Gillman, The Yellow Wallpaper, *1892*

An early example of American feminist literature, *The Yellow Wallpaper* is a searing portrayal of postpartum depression and the misogynistic attitudes towards it at the time. Locked up in a yellow-stained room, a woman descends into madness, as you generally would.

Henry James, Turn of the Screw, *1898*

When a young governess arrives at a crumbling mansion to look after two young children, she begins to suspect the ghosts of former servants are haunting them.

Aleister Crowley, Magick in Theory and Practice, *1912*

Drawing on a wide variety of sources, from yoga and medieval grimoires to Hermeticism and esotericists of the 19th century, *Magick in Theory and Practice* is a book of spells and occult theory for beginners from 20th-century sorcerer Aleister Crowley.

H P Lovecraft, The Dunwich Horror, *1928*

Purveyor of all things weird and wacky, H P Lovecraft was a prolific writer of ghoulish science fiction. *The Dunwich Horror* is the tale of Wilbur Whateley, a disfigured child who grows at an unnatural rate, and his even more sinister invisible twin brother.

Georges Bataille, Story of the Eye, *1928*

A disturbing story about a sexually depraved young couple and their penchant for shoving rounded objects (soft-boiled eggs, bull's testicles, a priest's eyeball) in a vast array of human orifices, *Story of the Eye* is a seminal work of Surrealist fiction.

Gerald Gardner, Book of Shadows, *c.1940*

Thought to have been created in the 40s by Gerald Gardner (the founder of the Neopagan religion Wicca, who claimed the sacred text was handed down to him by a powerful coven), the *Book of Shadows* is a set of instructions for magic rituals used within Wiccan communities today.

Anne Rice, Interview with the Vampire, *1976*

Told from the perspective of a hunky vampire with a human conscience, Louis de Pointe du Lac recounts his nefarious adventures with tyrannical creature of the night, Lestat.

Angela Carter, The Bloody Chamber, *1979*

Inspired by traditional fairy tales and folklore, *The Bloody Chamber and Other Stories* is a collection of short tales about a feral child, dismembered wives, an incestuous relationship with a fresh corpse and the malevolent Erl-King.

William Gibson, Neuromancer, *1984*
The book that essentially spawned the cyberpunk movement, William Gibson's *Neuromancer* is a sci-fi novel about a disgraced hacker in a dystopian underworld hired for one last dangerous job.

Kathy Acker, Empire of the Senseless, *1988*
A surreal sci-fi story about a cyborg named Abhor and her pirate love Thivai, and their iniquitous adventures involving prostitutes, terrorists and deranged doctors.

Propaganda Magazine, *1982–2002*
Founded by New York photographer Fred H Berger, *Propaganda Magazine* chronicled the saturnine style, music, art, literature and illicit sexploits of the American goth subculture from 1982 until 2002.

Bret Easton Ellis, American Psycho, *1991*
Patrick Bateman is a narcissistic Wall Street yuppie with an incredibly gothic self-care routine, whose increasing sense of alienation leads him into depravity.

Charlie Fox, This Young Monster, *2017*
Author and curator Charlie Fox pays homage to all things grisly and grotesque in his brilliant compendium of monsters through the ages.

Weird Walk, Weird Walk, 2023

A hauntological guide to Britain's ancient sites and mystic seasonal rituals, from cult zine creators and cultural phenomenon Weird Walk.

ART BOOKS

Like bats to a belfry, artists have been drawn to dark and alluring matter since, well, they've been drawn to art. And that's because art has the ability to shine a light on, and therefore make sense of, that lingering darkness within, whether the artist's own feelings of grief, terror, alienation, perversion, and/or angst, or those of another. From monographs on Hans Bellmer's deranged dolls to Arthur Jafa's brutalized Black bodies, here are some of the best art books to take with you to the grave.

Paris de Nuit, 1933

A bewitching black and white study of Paris under moonlight, French photographer Gilberte Brassaï captures the city's nocturnal revellers and their debauched escapades.

An Aperture Monograph, 1972

A love letter to freaks, misfits and fringe dwellers, Diane Arbus's *An Aperture Monograph* is an extensive survey of the photographer's haunting works.

The Family Album of Lucybelle Crater, *1974*
Southern gothic photographer Ralph Meatyard captures his wife, children and a rotating cast of characters dressed in grotesque rubber masks against a backdrop of American suburbia.

XXGirls, *1996*
Chronicler of America's dark underbelly and Cinema of Transgression daddy, Richard Kern's *XXGirls* comprises a series of black-and-white portraits of some pretty hardcore women, from Lydia Lunch to goth pin-up and actress Lung Leg with a lizard on her face.

Paul Delvaux: Surrealizing the Nude, *1992*
An examination of the nightmarish world of 20th-century artist Paul Delvaux and his morbid preoccupation with the nude.

Tokyo Love: Spring Fever, *1994*
Photographers Nan Goldin and Nobuyoshi Araki capture the underground club kids of 90s Tokyo and their niche sexual exploits.

Bob Flanagan: Supermasochist, *2000*
The late poet and performance artist Bob Flanagan made sadomasochistic work for sexual gratification. He also did it as a way to regain control over his ailing body, having been diagnosed with cystic fibrosis as a child. In his seminal book,

the artist welcomes you into his psychosexual arena and lays bare the intricate creative process behind his unique work.

Prints and Drawings of Käthe Kollwitz, 2000

An investigation into the maudlin works of German artist Käthe Kollwitz, who sought to come to terms with her son's death and the general sense of post-war suffering that dominated the period, through her monochromatic prints.

The Anatomy of Anxiety, 2002

An exhaustive study of controversial 20th-century artist Hans Bellmer, his convulsive images of dismembered dolls and their psychosexual origins.

The Cremaster Cycle, 2002

Published to coincide with a retrospective exhibition at the Guggenheim Museum, Matthew Barney's *The Cremaster Cycle* is a comprehensive study of the artist's surreal five-part film series in which he inhabits a slew of ghoulish roles including a satyr, magician and the infamous murderer Gary Gilmore. Combining interviews, essays and behind-the-scenes pictures, the book peels back the curtain on Barney's intricate process.

The Uncanny, 2004

An exploration of the uncanny through the creepy juxtaposition of mannequins and doll-like sculptures, this written companion to Kelly's 2004 exhibition at Tate

Liverpool explores the effects of memory, horror and anxiety on the human condition.

Surrealism, Alchemy and Art, *2004*
A definitive study of Mexican Surrealist artist Leonora Carrington and her fascination with dark fairy tales and the occult.

The Graphic Works of Odilon Redon, *2005*
Transforming everyday subjects into strange, fantastical beasts (spiders with human faces, one-eyed monsters and hairy fish), Symbolist artist Odilon Redon sought to recreate on canvas the dark complexities of his subconscious mind.

Drama and Theatre, *2018*
Accompanying an exhibition of Henry Fuseli's paintings at Basel's Kunstmuseum, *Drama and Theatre* explores the monstrous visions and dark romanticism of the renowned 18th-century British artist.

Love and Angst, *2019*
Though celebrated for his blood-curdling paintings of screaming figures, virgin-whores and creatures of the night, there's something inherently gothic about 19th-century Norwegian artist Edvard Munch's prints and their aching expressions of grief and misery, which were recently made the subject of a 2019 exhibition at the British Museum and its accompanying catalogue.

Magnumb, *2021*
Arthur Jafa's *Magnumb* explores the artist's stark portrayal of Black people living and suffering in America.

Walter Sickert, *2022*
Despite popular theories, there's zero evidence to suggest that Walter Sickert was actually Jack the Ripper. However, the artist reportedly did take an interest in East London's notorious serial killer, who would have dominated the headlines in 19th-century England – something that's evident in Sickert's voyeuristic depictions of sleeping nudes, which were shown as part of a recent retrospective at Tate Britain and in its accompanying catalogue.

Kara Walker: White Shadows in Blackface, *2023*
A survey of artist Kara Walker's eerie silhouettes and their representation of abject violence against African Americans, from antebellum time up to the modern day.

Chapter XV:
Undead men: goths to get out of the grave for

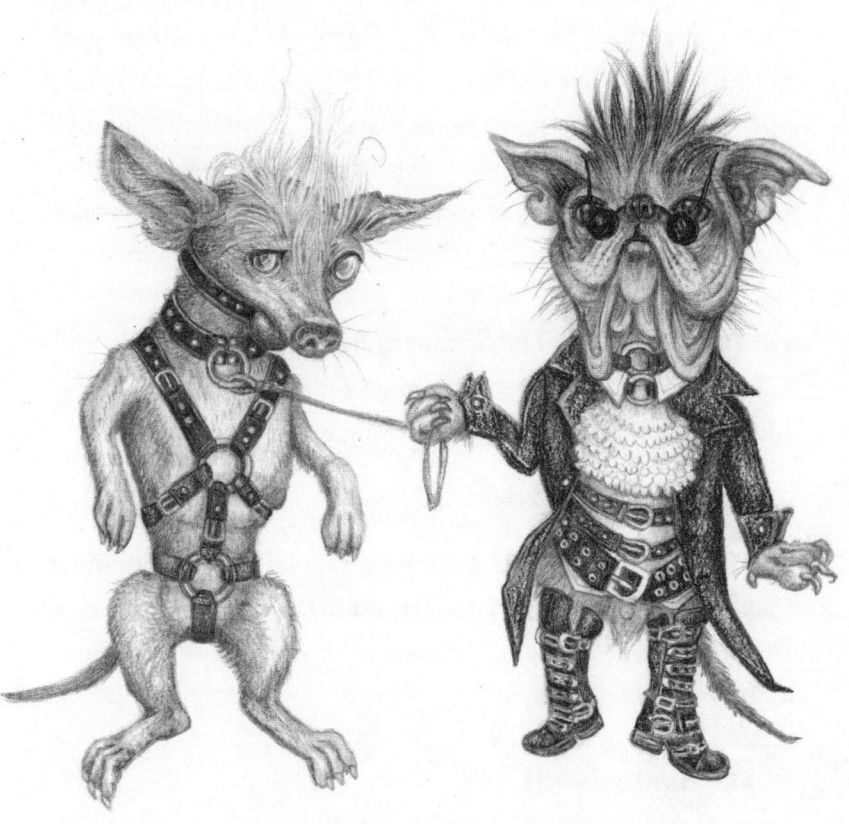

This book has been about women. So I thought we'd end with a few words on some maudlin men. Sad boys and goth geezers – the sort of chap who makes your pulse slow to a deadly beat. From Tim Burton's original misfit Edward Scissorhands, to Wesley Snipes's leather-clad vampire-hunter, Blade, sultry Swedish rapper Ecco2K to The Cure's Robert Smith, goth guys may seem to run the gamut of masculinity but generally speaking tend to be introspective, romantic and drawn to beauty and the macabre. As such, they make excellent bandmates, crypt fellows and companions with which to walk the earth.

Andrew Eldritch, *The Sisters of Mercy*
Charismatic frontman of wicked warblers The Sisters of Mercy. Expert lyricist who likes long graveyard walks.

Bela Lugosi
The 20th-century genre actor Bela Lugosi is best known for playing famed Transylvanian count in the 1931 horror classic *Dracula*. Has a very sexy Hungarian accent and looks great in a cape.

Blade, Blade (1998)
Masc for mac(acbre). Eligible bachelor number three is brooding vampire hunter Blade, played by Wesley Snipes. Into techno raves and slaying baddies; has his bloodlust somewhat under control.

Count Dracula, Bram Stoker's Dracula (1992)

If the crypt's a rockin', don't come a-knockin'. Immortalized by Gary Oldman, this European nobleman likes sanguine sports and carrying antique canes.

Dave Vanian, The Damned

A huge proponent of the 80s British goth scene, thanks to his vampiric get-up, lightning-streak hair and killer baritone. The Damned frontman has still got it, 40 years on.

Ecco2K

Swedish rapper and Drain Gang member, Ecco2K may look hard on the outside with his spooky makeup and layers of leather, but deep down he's just a sensitive soul.

Edward Scissorhands, Edward Scissorhands (1990)

Lonely heart looking for love, Edward Scissorhands likes horticulture, hairdressing and carving figures out of ice. Very good with his hands. Just don't invite him back to your water bed.

Eric Draven, The Crow (1994)

Tall, dark and recently brought back from the dead, Brandon Lee's Eric Draven likes big romantic gestures, sad clown makeup and the sweet taste of revenge.

Faris Badwan, *The Horrors*

With hair like the wings of a crow and a nose for the ages, The Horrors frontman Faris Badwan is your eligible bachelor number nine. Spends his days making art, writing songs and dressing as he did in the early noughties. He'll steal your skinny jeans, but you won't mind.

Frank N Furter, The Rocky Horror Picture Show *(1975)*

Mad scientist by day, freaky alien lover by night. Master dom looking for hunky sub to take to outer space.

Gomez Addams, The Addams Family *(1991)*

Cara mia. Family man looking for eternal companionship. Good with swords and severed hands. Demon in the sack. Will ravage you if you let him.

Lux Interior, *The Cramps*

Gothabilly daddy and The Cramps frontman Lux Interior likes roaming the streets at night, wearing head-to-toe leather and making a goo goo muck of things.

Ian Curtis, *Joy Division*

Run off into the afterlife with this international man of misery. Will love bomb you with his melancholy musings.

Morpheus, The Matrix *(1999)*

Teacher, leader, captain of his own ship, and deep down just a big ol' softie. Take the red pill with this one and never look back.

Peter Murphy, Bauhaus

Inky introvert and Bauhaus frontman Peter Murphy likes late-night séances, old-fashioned horror movies and trips up the belfry.

Nick Cave, Nick Cave and the Bad Seeds

Vampire to the Vampire's Wife, this diehard romantic is a fan of long-term commitments, power ballads and putting on a fresh suit. Will take things slow.

The Joker

Because sometimes, we all just want a bad boy who likes to watch the world burn. Big-time schemer, you can plot world domination with this one. Will laugh you into bed.

Robert Smith, The Cure

This prince of darkness likes long strolls in the forest and playing the guitar. Very good with words. Might steal your lipstick.

Vincent Price

Horror hunk Vincent Price is the stuff of Hollywood legend. Great with ghosts, monsters and wax figures. Knows his way around a haunted house. Fun fact: his grandfather invented tartar-based baking powder.

Yung Lean

Let Swedish rapper and ultimate sad boy Yung Lean take you to (Sound)cloud nine and serenade you with his syrupy music and melancholy vocals.

Yves Tumor

Yves Tumor makes spooky songs for spooky people. Likes scaring the mainstream and looks great in a wig.

Chapter XVI:
The future is goth

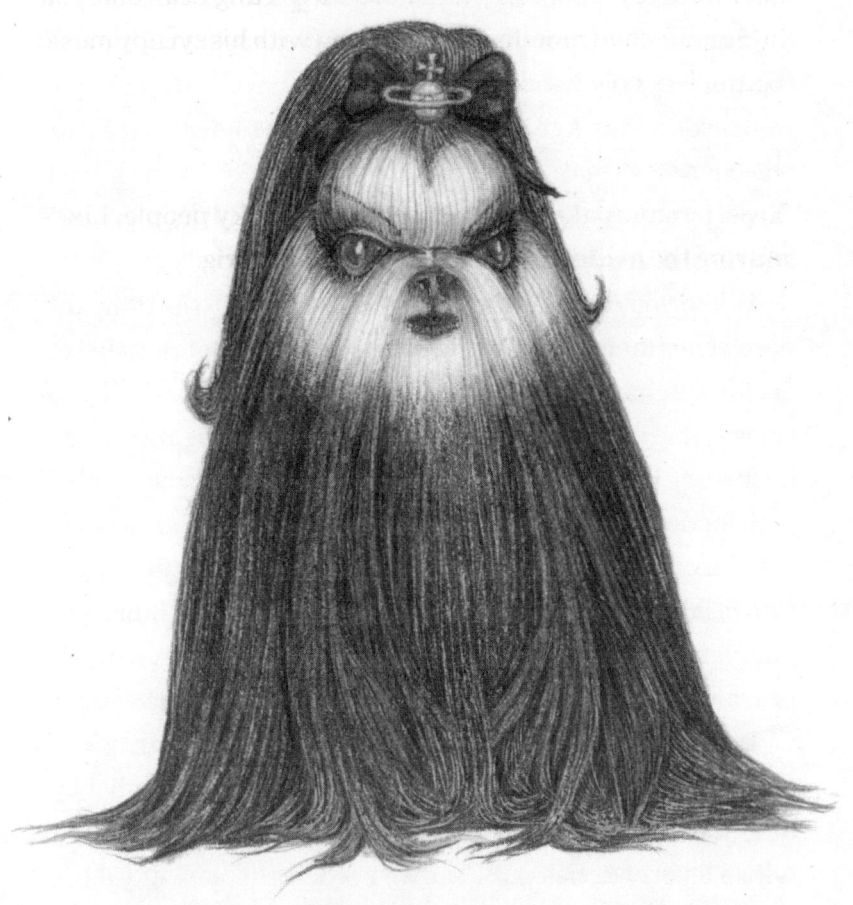

We've seen where goth has been, but what about where it's heading? Picture any imagined rendering of the future from the last century or so – whether in art, music, fashion or film – there's always something Giger-esque about it, a dystopian vision filled with monsters, aliens and humanoid hybrids living on a planet on the brink of self-destruction. Think of the horror-stricken ramblings of H P Lovecraft, Stanley Kubrick's Space Age cacotopias, Thierry Mugler's autumn/winter 1995 cyborg suit (worn in February 2024 on the red carpet by actress Zendaya to the premiere of sci-fi movie *Dune*) and most of Arca's visual output.

When you combine the horrors of today with the rampant pace of technological advancements and the looming threat of climate change, it's not beyond the realms of possibility to suggest that we are hurtling towards an apocalypse and there's no turning back. But these are conditions in which the humble goth tends to flourish. Where others see darkness and doom, we see romance and possibility. In fact, the very notion of the future is at its core incredibly goth. Which is why, a hundred-plus years from now, the state of being goth will be even more prevalent – as a necessary way to cope with all the madness.

But there's something else happening here too. Intrinsic to the goth experience is the idea of being an outsider, whether by design or default. And because of that, goths are still viewed with a level of derision. But as we become increasingly more inclusive and accepting of perceived differences, I predict that those who identify outside the prescribed norms will be given even more space to thrive, with the state of being goth being embraced by an even wider audience. Furthermore, the very notion of the outsider will become normalized, meaning that those who have an urgent need to subvert and rebel will have to push the boundaries even further than before. But it also means that others will be free to be themselves without having to push any boundaries at all.

So what will the goths of tomorrow actually look like? As creatures of the night increasingly base their beauty choices on a pick and mix of references, the goth aesthetic will become even more fluid, a composite of extreme iterations of individualism. At one end of the beauty spectrum, the shock tactics of the 80s and 90s goths, as well as contemporary beauty mavericks Fecal Matter, Doja Cat and Michèle Lamy, will become even more subversive. But there will also be a contingency of inky fiends who eschew makeup altogether. It's a similar story for style: monstrous silhouettes and hardcore industrial materials at one end and a more normcore proposition at the other, perhaps with a predilection for fabrics that respond to the outside elements. It's giving functional futuristic goth. And this is the case for goths at any stage of life, particularly as lives become even longer. Which brings me to self-care. With increasing importance being placed on health and wellbeing, biohacking will become integral to the goth experience. Think robotic limbs, everyday transplants and strange wellness methods that have yet to be invented. But above all, the language of goth will be just another way of expressing your true self, whoever that might be. As such, the possibilities are endless and, above all, thrilling. Which can only mean one thing: the season of the witch is far from over.

Long live the goth.

Afterword

Fecal Matter: on provoking society

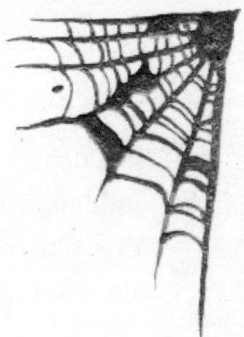

Ignore the stares, ignore the fear. Set yourself free. Release yourself from the constraints of normality. Shed your anxiety, live your truth and take control. Don't let them abuse you. Provoke society, elevate humanity. Provoke society, just live your truth.

Individuals like us who stand out are subjected to ridicule, violence, hatred and judgement on a daily basis. Not only on the streets or on the bus, but often in our homes and by our families. Sometimes it can feel like there are no safe spaces to exist in.

Standing out and being yourself forces people to step outside of their comfort zones and think critically, which can trigger polarizing reactions. This can make one feel alienated and alone, almost like an unwanted alien; but it can also bring people together when you discover others who share the same daily path to freedom.

During our hard times in public, when people are pointing and laughing, when there is danger coming our way, the 'provoke society' mantra helps us walk through the fire. It reminds us to live fearlessly.

Acknowledgements

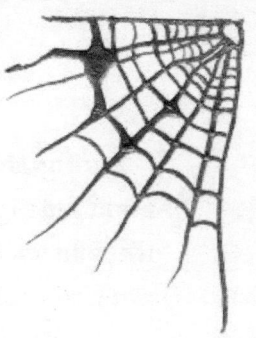

And now for a few words of thanks to those without whom this would not have been possible: my family and friends for putting up with me throughout this whole process; my publisher, editors, subeditors, Briony Gowlett and Rimsha Falak for making this happen and making it the best it can be; Elise Solberg for persuading me to do this; Aurel Schmidt for bringing my words to life via her brilliant illustrations; Indigo Lewin, Hikari Yokoyama, Alex Peters and Charlie Fox for their sage advice; a huge thank you to Mert Alas for capturing me at my most gothic on the back cover; and to Hanna Hanra for her wisdom, Amanda Harlech for her eloquence and Fecal Matter for being themselves. I'm so grateful for everyone who has worked on this book, to the wondrous muses who inspired it and to everyone who answered my calls and emails and gave up their time to contribute. To all the goths that have come before me and all that will come after. And to my husband Tom, the Gomez to my Morticia, the light to all my darkness, a lifetime of thank yous.

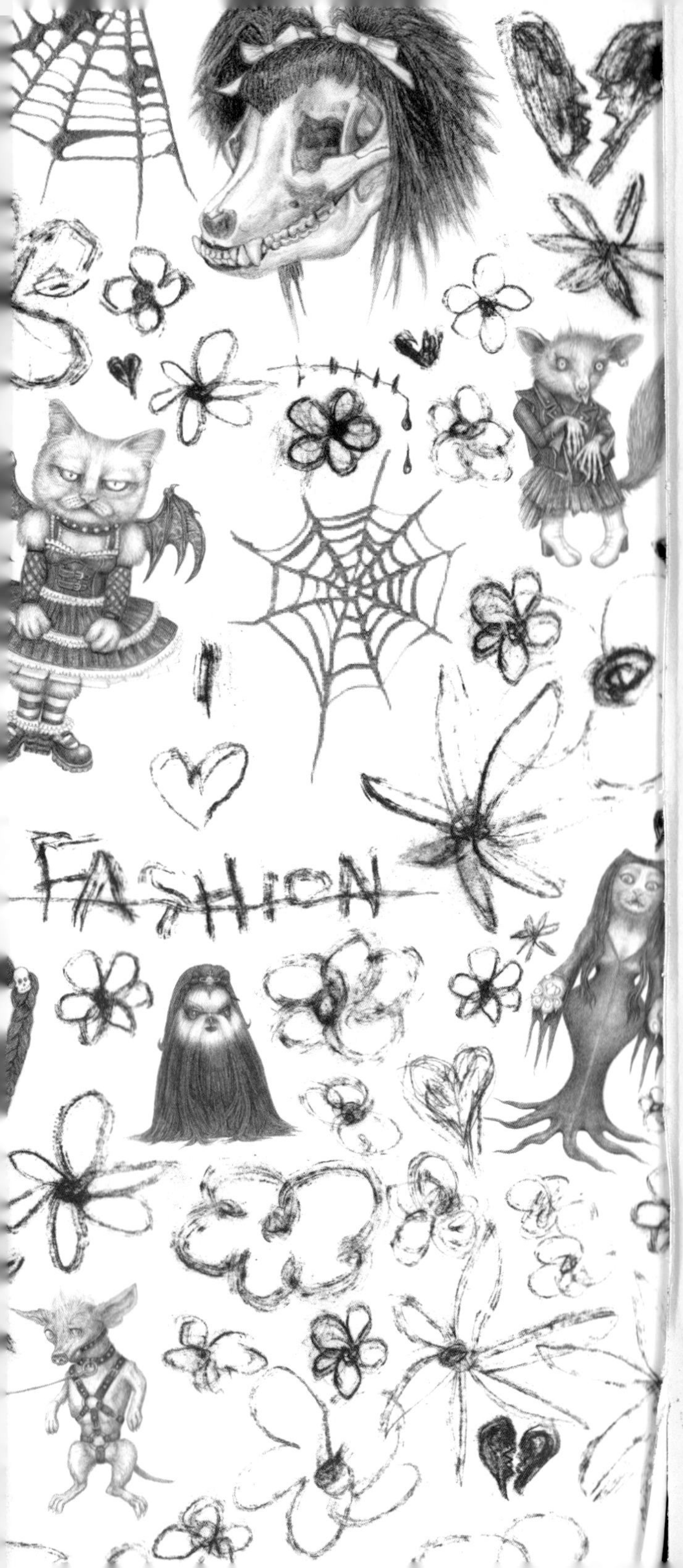

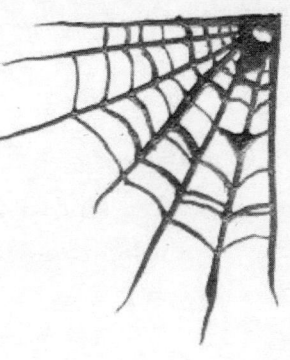

About the author

Tish Weinstock is a London-based writer, editor and consultant specialising in beauty and its intersection with fashion, lifestyle and pop culture.

Graduating from Oxford University in 2012 with a degree in History of Art, she has worked at style bibles *i-D*, *Dazed & Confused* and *British Vogue*, where she remains Contributing Beauty Editor. In 2022, she joined *System* magazine as Beauty Director to launch its sister title *System Beauty*. She also contributes to *The Week*, *Sunday Times Style*, *Pop Magazine*, *AnOther* and *Arena Homme +*.